"Weighty in content and graphic in description, Harold Burchett chronicles his pilgrimage from senior pastor to full-time caregiver of his Alzheimer-afflicted wife, Jane. Intensely personal and at times painfully vulnerable, *Last Light* provides both highly practical advice and ~~ ~
spiritual counsel centered in the cross of Christ. This is ~ ¹
caregivers of Alzheimer victims, but also ⸁
entrusted with the long-term care of a lo

—K⸜
Columbia Biblical S

"In recent years, the world has been treated ⸜ᴧι moving memoirs written by authors whose spouses suffer from Alzheimer's. Harold Burchett's contribution to this literature is unusual for several reasons. Most notable is the edifying Christian reflection that the disease has prompted. But almost as notable is the great honesty Burchett displays in describing the human trauma—but also the beauty of human tenderness—that the disease has brought. It is a moving account of 'bearing the cross,' but also being borne by the Savior of the Cross."

—MARK NOLL, PROFESSOR OF HISTORY,
Wheaton College

"From his heart, and in his unique style, Harold Burchett discards conventional dignity, and with tender frankness, captures the embarrassment, the heartbreak, the helplessness, and even the comical, that confronts the caregiver of a beloved spouse. The ultimate victory of the Cross—turning terminal tragedy into triumph and thus finding 'strength in God alone'—breathes the encouragement of a modern-day Psalm."

—GORDON E. STIMERS, PASTORAL CARE,
High Park Baptist Church, Toronto Canada

"*Last Light*, by Harold (and Jane) Burchett, is the love story of two remarkable Christians. As a young teenager, I came to know that my pastor and his spouse were godly persons who did not want to miss one lesson from God . . . or one occasion to grow to be more like Jesus. Now in the waning years of Jane's Alzheimer's, Harold has given us an honest, sad, thoughtful, and hopeful account. God will continue to prophetically use Jane and Harold to strengthen, encourage, and comfort the church of Jesus Christ."

—DR. ART GAY, PASTOR,
First Baptist Church, Portland, Maine

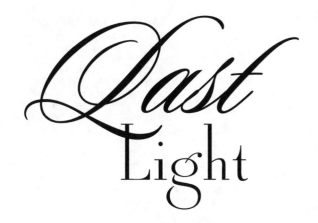

Last
Light

Staying True Through
the Darkness of Alzheimer's

HAROLD E. BURCHETT
Foreword by Robertson McQuilkin

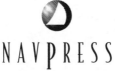

NAVPRESS

Bringing Truth to Life
P.O. Box 35001, Colorado Springs, Colorado 80935

The Navigators is an international Christian organization. Our mission is to reach, disciple, and equip people to know Christ and to make Him known through successive generations. We envision multitudes of diverse people in the United States and every other nation who have a passionate love for Christ, live a lifestyle of sharing Christ's love, and multiply spiritual laborers among those without Christ.

NavPress is the publishing ministry of The Navigators. NavPress publications help believers learn biblical truth and apply what they learn to their lives and ministries. Our mission is to stimulate spiritual formation among our readers.

© 2002 by Harold E. Burchett
All rights reserved. No part of this publication may be reproduced in any form without written permission from NavPress, P.O. Box 35001, Colorado Springs, CO 80935.
www.navpress.com

Library of Congress Catalog Card Number: 2001052106
ISBN 1-57683-298-8

Cover design by Dan Jamison
Cover photo by ROB & SAS / The Stock Market
Creative Team: Lori Mitchell, Anita Palmer, Amy Spencer, Glynese Northam

Unless otherwise identified, all Scripture quotations in this publication are taken from the HOLY BIBLE: NEW INTERNATIONAL VERSION® (NIV®). Copyright © 1973, 1978, 1984 by International Bible Society. Used by permission of Zondervan Publishing House. All rights reserved.

Burchett, Harold Ewing.
    Last light : staying true through the darkness of alzheimer's / Harold E. Burchett.
        p. cm.
    ISBN 1-57683-298-8
    1. Caregivers--Biography. 2. Spouses of clergy--Biography. 3. Alzheimer's disease--Patients--Biography. 4. Alzheimer's disease--Patients--Family relationships--Biography. I. Title.

RC523.2 .B87 2002
362.1'96831--dc21   2001052106

Printed in the United States of America
1 2 3 4 5 6 7 8 9 10 / 06 05 04 03 02

FOR A FREE CATALOG OF
NAVPRESS BOOKS & BIBLE STUDIES,
CALL 1-800-366-7788 (USA)
OR 1-416-499-4615 (CANADA)

Contents

Foreword

Astonishing! That's the best word I know to express the impact Harold Burchett has had on hundreds of pastors and missionaries. But maybe even more on laypeople. I'll never forget the first Saturday morning I attended his men's discipleship session in the church he pastored—seventy men giving up Saturday morning to get pummeled with Harold's flat-out brand of discipleship. And it was no fluke. Twenty-five years later I attended a similar Saturday morning session in another church he had just begun to pastor. Why would these fifty men keep coming back for more? Because their lives were being transformed! But when it came his turn, would it work? Would the counsel of the master disciplemaker deliver him from evil?

At the summit of his pastoral ministry, Burchett's energetic lifelong partner in ministry began to fall victim to Alzheimer's disease. Or was it the reluctant caregiver who was victim? You have here the story of one man's struggle with saying "the long good-bye" to his beloved.

The author is nothing if not a private person, yet here he opens the door and invites you in to feel the pain, to watch the stumbles. But also to witness God's deliverances, small and great. You will weep. But you will exult in the bright hope that shines through the dark nights of our lives. In this little book you will find practical help for the challenges of giving and accepting care. But much more: you will find a story of beauty and grace birthed in agony and loss.

ROBERTSON MCQUILKIN,
PRESIDENT EMERITUS AT COLUMBIA (S.C.) INTERNATIONAL UNIVERSITY
AND AUTHOR OF *A PROMISE KEPT*, AN ALZHEIMER'S LOVE STORY.

Acknowledgments

Among the good friends who held back the clouds so I could record this story are Robertson McQuilkin, who helped me better understand Alzheimer's; Bob and Mary Ann Sandefur, who provided office space in their home and much assistance to Jane and me; all those who regularly lifted our loads; and our family, for their steady encouragement. Finally, Craig Noll and Anita Palmer gave invaluable professional help in improving the manuscript.

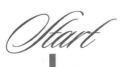

Squeezed into Life

> *"One day when you are old, you will be forced to change—you'll see!"*
>
> —JANE, A PROPHECY EARLY IN OUR MARRIAGE

YEARS AGO I ONCE TEASED MY WIFE, JANE, THAT SHE SHOULD PROPOSE anew to me on bended knee. Little did I realize that one day—like Joseph's brothers—I would kneel before her every day for years! In daily dressing and undressing, bathing, and other caregiving duties requiring kneeling at her feet, I have found myself there hundreds and hundreds of times.

Early in our marriage Jane startled me once by answering one of my forceful and finely put arguments with a kind of prophecy: "One day when you are old, you will be forced to change—*you'll see!*" Though we never referred to these words again, instantly I knew they were spoken in the Spirit. This book is a recounting of how all has been (and is being) fulfilled. As Jane predicted, I am now not what I was. By the mercy of God, my intense involvement with Jane's Alzheimer's disease has not squeezed life out of me. It has squeezed life in.

Sadly, this narration reports also the last light of an organized, able leader among women, to the point where she is unable to make a bed or care for her own personal needs. The family champion at speed word games cannot now spell or write her own name or read. Her three-under-par miniature golf score, even with early Alzheimer's, was good enough to beat family and friends, but now she is pathetically dependent on us all.

What God has taught me in the College of Dementia Caregiving about his love and power in the face of insurmountable heartbreak is not just applicable to Alzheimer's. It applies also to anyone facing the fall-out of drug addiction, cancer, loneliness, broken families, or a myriad of life's trials.

Any family members who take on the task of caregiving will understand at the outset that theirs is a war they must fight knowing all the while they cannot win. Day by day they are forced to renew the battle, which is inevitably lost day by day. Never is there to be any lasting progress. Here, then, is the marvel of the Christian caregiver's faith. While he or she seems to be losing all, that caregiver is yet winning. Losing inches, yet winning by miles. From this divine point of view, it is better to win while losing than to lose while winning.

This process that I call "winning" has no place for forced, dry-as-dust religious clichés. No such thinking can survive long in the arena where the champion of dementia holds forth.

CHOOSING TO LOSE

Sometime after the neurologist pronounced over our two heads what we accept as the plan of providence for our lives, I asked Jane, "Honey, if you could have your wish, would you choose to go back like we were before the Alzheimer's, or would you rather have our relationship like it is now and have the sickness?" Without a moment's hesitation, she said, "I like it the way things are now." I agreed—and still do. We have had a good marriage that has lasted half a century, but there is a new tender caring between us now that is beyond anything we ever dreamed of in earlier years.

As you will see in the first chapter, Jane and I—even before we realized what was happening—were being pulled into a tunnel that is dark and very long. The beginning of our now ceaseless struggle is chronicled there.

The next several chapters are to provide some insight and perspective on life with one who has dementia. A day out of my diary (chapter 2) reveals the depth to which life is changed. Communicating with Jane requires a new language, one that alters daily (chapter 3). I try in chapter 4 to illustrate the only way I have found to endure these changing trials through the love nurtured by God himself. He is powerfully present, even in the withering experiences I narrate in chapter 5. Because of his presence I can recount in chapter 6 the sustaining humor that leavens the trauma. And in chapter 7, written particularly for those who are shouldering caregiving responsibilities, I list practical suggestions for tending the ill.

Once the storm front of these intense experiences began to clear, truths that I had known generally for years stood forth for me to grasp in a new and very personal way. Insights came with special clarity and perspective. Lessons from the agony (chapter 8) have led to insight (chapter 9). Suffering has helped seeing.

CHASING THE SETTING SUN

The thought of never again hearing Jane pray or of never again receiving any of her penetrating words of correction and encouragement was so unbearable to me that years ago I began making hasty notes as she would sometimes unexpectedly pray or challenge me spiritually. Armed with notepads strategically placed about the house, I wrote as things occurred, sometimes with tears during the more painful incidents. In hopes of preserving the light in her words, and with a desire to share what

I learned standing in that light, I have written this book.

To read the prayers and prophecies of an Alzheimer's patient will perhaps seem surprising. They astounded me each time they came, and I am so glad now that I made the effort to record them. Chapter 10, then, is "Jane's Prayers and Prophecies." These rays of light occasionally flashing from Jane's spirit were to me glimpses of her last light, which has given title to this book. "My Confessions and Tribute to Jane" is my finish to this story.

HESITATIONS . . . AND A PRAYER FOR YOU, THE READER

Before this writing, I penned a small booklet addressed to our neighbors, introducing Jane and me and explaining why the two of us live in such apparent hibernation. I gave these out door to door, person to person, to many scores of our neighbors as a testimony to God's saving and sustaining kindness. The response was more than I could have hoped.

Friends who heard me over recent years state that I would never write about these experiences might be surprised to learn that I wrote the booklet and, even more, that I am writing this book. Why had I recorded all these events, even actual words spoken? I cannot fully explain why, other than by saying that some of the experiences were extremely powerful and dear to me; without writing them down in some way, my overtaxed brain was in danger of losing them all in the course of each day's confusion. A few notes or pages here and there over months and years added up to a large file. Gradually, I came to feel that I should write a more complete account than just the booklet, not so much of the chronology of Jane's illness as of the light observed and lessons learned. You are now holding this account.

Before launching, I must confess my dread in divulging all that you are about to read. Will our defeats and dark struggles

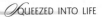

spread darkness? (And darkness is contagious.) But there is another dread: when triumphs are celebrated, will they weigh down on those who find no rainbow in their clouds? May God—the God even of these hesitations—bring helpful instruction, new insights, and only encouragement!

Entering the Dark Tunnel

"Well, you see I am not falling apart."

—JANE, ON HEARING THE
DOCTOR'S DIAGNOSIS

RUSHING TO ITS FEARFUL DESTINATION, THE DREADED TRAIN PASSED OUR way. Against our will, my wife and I were hauled aboard and are now being forced to pay for the ride again and again. That is how it is with Alzheimer's.

Married couples who have pledged to stand together until death parts them know that at some time all husbands and wives must enter the dark tunnel and experience that parting. But I never expected the tunnel to be so long and so dark, or the parting to be so continuous! Each new day I go to the cemetery and leave there another part of my wife of nearly fifty years. That is how it seems. Try as I might, I can't stop the process. It goes on and on and on, as it has for ten years.

SLOWLY IT DAWNED: "IT'S GETTING DARK!"

More than eight years ago, Jane began having difficulty with our friends, and especially with me. This experience tossed me into a period of soul-searching. Was I troubling our marriage? No, it wasn't that (though I could be difficult at times!). Jane was changing. It seemed as though something was wrong with her mind. Reality was sometimes confused with fears and imagination, and her memory was failing noticeably. This situation left her agitated and at times angry. Not knowing what the developing dementia was doing to her mind, Jane assumed that people around her were fouled up.

For about a year, I joined Jane in thrashing about in this unexplainable turmoil. Slowly, however, the dark truth became clear. My strong and steady life partner was becoming unstable and unpredictable. I finally concluded that it had to be Alzheimer's or some other form of dementia.

THEN I WENT UNDERGROUND

Any suggestion that the problem was hers put Jane on the defense (or the offense!). In this early stage, I felt guilty even at the thought of telling our two sons and two daughters that something was wrong with their mother. Furthermore, I was then senior pastor of a very active church in Virginia Beach, Virginia, and we were just getting nicely settled into the ministry. How could I tell the people that their pastor's wife was afflicted with dementia? I'll just sit on the problem until I know what to do, I reasoned.

But how do you hide Alzheimer's? Relentlessly, its grip tightened. Names of friends went first from Jane's memory. Soon even family members could not be recalled by name. As months passed, she lost her ability to read and write, to tell time, to remember the day, month, or year, or even to say where we live.

Alterations in the routines of our lives were coming fast. Jane must not drive anymore. Changes came in household and personal matters. Decisions had to be made. Then came the medical and psychological testing that confirmed my fears.

On a Friday, our neurologist asked to see us, but I was to come alone first. "I wish I could tell you that your wife has a brain tumor," he began. Hearing the diagnosis — "Alzheimer's" — both shook me and relieved me. All worrisome wondering was over, but a numb grief, followed by a giant loneliness, wrapped me in its shadows as I walked to my car. I turned on the ignition and the radio came on. Amazingly, a voice from the radio spoke these very words from 2 Corinthians 12:9: "My grace is sufficient for you, for my power is made perfect in weakness."

Next I brought Jane into the doctor's office, and we sat side by side in front of his desk. As kindly as he could, he informed her. All she said was, "Well, you see I am not falling apart."

Outside, I proposed that we not think or talk but go get an ice cream instead. Then we spent the rest of that Friday and Saturday weeping. Literally our tears pooled together as we held one another. All thoughts of being brave were over-whelmed by our anguish over what we were to endure and what we were losing. Words no longer worked. We just cried with each other before God.

GOING PUBLIC

Then we began to function. The family was told everything. But what about the church? Jane decided to tell the congregation herself, publicly. I encouraged her. By now Sunday was upon us, and I chose to speak on Psalm 84, using the simple theme of trusting in God. I think God helped me through it. Then I added these words, "Jane and I soon will have been married forty-five years. As many of you know, she has been undergoing medical tests. She is here to tell you personally of the results, because what we heard from the doctor was heavy, very heavy indeed."

Standing at the pulpit, Jane opened with a simple poem she had selected bearing the theme "He holds my hand." Her next words brought many audible gasps and sobs from our dear church friends.

> A little more than forty hours ago, Harold and I sat in the doctor's office to get the report on all the tests. Already we have told our four children. Now I want you to know. The doctors say I have the beginning of Alzheimer's disease. We need your prayers as we prepare for difficult days. I love you all. Thank you.

The outpouring of hugs and tearful words of encouragement immediately and forever erased any doubt about going public so early. Now we could set ourselves to figure out how to cope. Shadows were already gathering at a fearful rate.

STAGGERING BUT STILL STANDING

The next months became a blur of mixed staggering and standing. Having never done much in the way of household duties and still less of serious caregiving, I staggered from one day to the next as these responsibilities claimed an ever-increasing amount of my time. Much practical assistance from the church, including three hot meals a week delivered to our table, enabled me to continue active ministry for four more years. But there was a heavy price.

Without warning or preparation, I was being ushered into new experiences, such as choosing my wife's clothing for each day and, eventually, having to dress her. As time went on, bathing, as well as dental and toilet care, then became my responsibilities. Often these tasks were made excruciatingly tedious by Jane's stubborn refusal to cooperate. "What do you know about these things?" she would demand, to which I would respond, "But you can't go out like that; you haven't finished dressing!" or "No, you can't wear that in the bath!"

How does one go about brushing another's teeth, especially

when that one adamantly says no? Someone should write a book on how to do that task, being sure to include a few lines on how to get the dentures out and then back in when the "victim" insists that she has no such thing as a "tenure" or a "pate of teef" in her mouth.

Meaningful communication becomes increasingly difficult as a loved one hears you say what you did not say and forgets what she has just said. For example, "Harold, please come and sit here; listen, it's important."

"Okay, what is it?"

"Uh, well, you know, don't you? I forget."

"That's okay. We'll think of it later."

Often "hot" meant "cold," and "strong" indicated "long" or "big" or "heavy." Even her "no, no" often meant "okay." The names of colors were forgotten or interchanged. I came to see that the loss of memory was invading every dimension of life. Unrelentingly, this specter reached especially into areas of relationship, devouring everything.

Earlier, while she was still able to schedule medical appointments for herself, considerable difficulties arose from her unexpected cancellations, confusion of dates, and suspicions of those in charge of her treatment. Once a concern turned to worry, paranoia was sure to follow.

I felt I had to make a daily, hour-by-hour effort to hold open the closing door of Jane's memory bank, but I continued to lose the battle. At this writing, the past is almost erased. Now the eraser swipes out the past five minutes, or even closer. A special restaurant meal is forgotten before we arrive home: "I'm hungry; could we get something to eat?" is the regular theme of our return trip. (Before this book was finished, Jane's memory span could not support even a brief sentence; after uttering several words, she no longer could recall what she started out to say. Now much of the time she gives out a stream of disconnected, meaningless words and phrases, or only sounds.)

WHICH WAY IS UP—DOES ANYBODY KNOW?

Mixed in the swirl of confusing developments were my own years of training and experience in teaching and counseling others. Home now provided a humbling contrast. I no longer sat in calm charge of everything. Instead, I longed for an 800 number to some customer service where I might appeal, "Anybody there know which way is up in my latest crisis?" Being locked in all these experiences with Alzheimer's trimmed me down—from feeling "professional" to "puny."

Utter devastation. Often I was like a lonely survivor of an intense bombing raid climbing out from a crater, asking, "What hit me?" Even this question I had to amend to, "What's going to hit me next?" because inevitably I could hear the "bombers" returning for another round.

Precisely right there was the big test, that of getting up again from the overwhelmingness to face yet more absolute impossibilities. Of not abandoning hope, though I knew the situation would only worsen and could never improve. Concerning his great burden as a gospel herald, the apostle Paul once asked, "And who is equal to such a task?" Then he answered his own question, "Our competence comes from God" (2 Corinthians 2:16; 3:5).

To give the reader an idea of what Jane's disease presents, I list here a sampling of experiences regularly faced in the years before the final phase, which brings a more complete loss of intelligent speech and of physical mobility.

- Unable to get her own cup of tea, even with help.
- Carrying frozen food from the refrigerator about the house.
- Endless questions, repeated and re-repeated: "How old am I?" "What time is it?" "What day is this?" "Where do we live?" "Is this our home?" "Where are you?" Often said when I'm within sight, if not reach: "Are you still here?" Spoken with anxiety: "Is everything all right?" "Am I doing

something wrong?" (This last question pains me, and I keep trying to release her from carrying such concern.)

- Clutter collecting and clutter carrying. This habit has continued into the disease's more advanced form, though not as intensely as at first. Both hands and arms are loaded with stuffed animals, clothing, shoes, paper towels and napkins, postcards, photos, personal mail new or old, colorful scraps of paper or cloth or plastic, clothespins, bobby pins, curlers, magazines, dish towels, placemats, much of which she dutifully carries throughout the day. Having to unload her arms for meals, for each trip to the bathroom, for going anyplace outside, or when dressing and undressing is no small challenge. Every night before retiring, she carefully arranges her belongings on the bed—up to twenty articles—all in a definite pattern. I have learned that if I don't protest this inconvenience but rather show respect for these things she values, then she will allow me to stack them nearby, until she begins another day carrying about what I have not in the meanwhile hidden or smuggled out to the trash barrel.
- Eating the dog's food.
- Problems with clothing, such as wearing a woolen sweater in sweltering heat, climbing into bed fully clothed and resisting any pressure to change, or making an appearance before guests or even in public not fully clothed.
- Losing things regularly. This problem sets up some unusual search expeditions, if she helps. "Now, what is it we are looking for?" Followed by, "Is this it?" as she produces a wide assortment of unrelated items.
- Accomplishing anything out of the house such as shopping or dining—any activity that involves the unsuspecting public provides endless challenges, humor, and embarrassment.

MY "NEVER-AGAINS"

With a strong finality it dawned on me that many precious experiences would never again be part of our lives. Vacations. Even a day off. A meal prepared and served by Jane. Or any further use of our dinnerware, at least in a proper manner. Holding a garage sale brought a peculiar sadness—as if I were a grieving widower breaking up the home.

In the dark tunnel, Alzheimer's strong arm begins immediately to destroy every vestige of hope and sanity if self-pity comes along for the ride. My way of coping is to pray and refocus on Jane's need. Often I have looked into her anxious eyes and promised as I did at the wedding altar (this time with tears and many years of growing up), "Jane, you are the dearest on earth to me, and with God helping me, I will never, ever leave or fail you."*

---

* This commitment, of course, involves doing what is best for the patient, not what is simply agreeable. I want very much to fulfill my vows to Jane by caring for her at home, but it will depend on my continued physical strength. So far, except for a brief try-out of day care, I have been able to weather each new phase without institutional help. Though it is an answer in some cases, I determined that such an arrangement was not for us.

Diary of a Day

"When will we be getting something ready to eat?"

—JANE, SHORTLY AFTER ARRIVING HOME

FROM A CAFETERIA MEAL

FEELING A NEED TO GAIN PERSPECTIVE, I ONCE MADE THE DECISION TO record a day in the life of Harold and Jane to share with our children and a few friends. It took hours of work to get an entire day down on paper, but I did it. The day selected was Monday, July 6, 1998, some three years before the writing of this book, so the disease was in a milder state and the days less trying. Also, I had not yet resigned as pastor of the church. Here is an excerpt of the actual diary entry, followed by some thoughts and reflections.

8:00 A.M. Today is our regular day off, and I decide to sleep in a little. Jane gets up early (usually I'm up first). The sound of her taking out her pills awakens me with a jolt. "Honey, where did you get the medicine?" Apparently, she has gotten into the main supply of her heart medicine, which I have hidden in order to monitor dosages.

Daily confusion over the morning newspaper. "Come, see what is out front!" Next, two problems: (1) making sure I see the paper before it disappears into the trash and (2) hiding or disposing of its plastic bag and any attractive circulars therein before Jane possesses them as treasures to be saved. One confiscated flier reappears on the couch, so I repossess it.

By now I realize I'll have no personal prayer and Bible study this day until after breakfast.

Next ritual, get hot water and soap in the dishpan and try to offset her only rinsing dishes and silverware under the cold tap water. She washes them at various times during meals, so I must get ahead of her and be alert for any sticky or greasy tableware.

Hearing water running when we're eating, she invariably asks, "What is going on?" I explain in such a way to keep her at the table. This morning I help her squeeze her grapefruit and catch the juice.

Phone rings. I'm informed an acquaintance has just died. I explain the identity of the deceased: "Remember, yesterday we visited the dying person at the hospital." She's not sure.

I take out the trash. Garbage and kitchen waste is of little concern to her, but she is ever anxious over certain containers, plastic bags, or shiny promotional circulars. This time I slip in everything without protest from her, though she follows me out to the recycle barrel.

I rescue today's paper and get her to yield up a stack of napkins and paper towels she is carrying. (We go through rolls and stacks of paper products at an unbelievable rate.)

As I pass the bedroom door, I hear, "Who bumped up all this?" Interpretation: "The bedding is unusually messed up." At this stage of the disease she can put the bed into a passable condition, but I must change linens and do the laundry.

9:00 A.M. My writing this narrative is interrupted by her call. Can't locate her clothes. A few moments later my Bible study is interrupted. She appears with a slip on lower half, but on upper body has good Sunday blouse and heavy winter blazer. It's a hot summer day. I make the mistake of giving more than one suggestion. Her response tells me nothing was communicated or accepted. I return to my office, to let it play out or whatever.

I have not had the opportunity to dress. She comes to the bathroom door several times—as she always does—asking, "Are you okay? Can I help you?" On entering the bedroom, I recognize some cards I had earlier thrown into the recycle bin. When I remonstrate, she smiles and gives me a hearty raspberry. As she inhales for a second blast, I press the cards over her mouth. This creates an explosion, and we both laugh.

Next she wants to show me a special little box of jewelry. "Do you remember these? Very valuable and special." (Showed them to me last night, as she often does.) "Somebody gave to me." I remind her that I gave them to her. "Yes," she says.

10:00 A.M. For a few precious minutes she plays the piano until she hears me going through the family room. I'm on my way to attempt a patch job on two pillowcases that I retrieved from the trash barrel the other day. They match bed linen but need stitching. Not knowing how to do that, I'm trying cloth cement, laying out the job on the breakfast table, under a couple of books. I invite Jane to sit and observe so she won't move it before it dries. Later I clean up the clutter and lay the pillowcases aside for the next laundry. I'm putting this off until the professional cleaners come to do the house in a few days. They also change the bed sheets. That is difficult for me to do, with Jane's "help." (Incidentally, all my cementing efforts went down the laundry drain; the cement washed away.)

Must get ladder to climb into the attic and check on a problem there. "What in the world are you doing?" Jane calls from the bottom of the ladder. All the while I'm up there, her warnings and admonitions continue. I finish and put away the ladder. Periodically, she forgets where I am and comes calling, "Are you still there?" or "Where are you?"

Noon. As we leave for lunch, she begins asking, "Where we going?" Though the cafeteria name is familiar to her and she passes it daily, she really can't recall it. So all along the way, the name must be repeated patiently.

As always, Jane dresses for anticipated cold weather outside, though it's in the eighties or nineties. She becomes very agitated if I say something like, "You can't wear your winter jacket—it's blazing hot out there." "What do you mean, I can't? You are dressed, aren't you?" "Okay, bring it along."

As we enter the garage I say, "See how hot it is? Give me the jacket and I'll keep it in the car for you." I am grateful she puts down the extra pairs of shoes she often carries, but she still has a fistful of paper towels, napkins, and ever-present safety pins.

"While I back out the car, would you please take this bag of trash to the black barrel?" "Where?" "Outside that door," pointing to the garage side door. "But how?" "Go around outside, there." "Okay."

She returns, still holding the bag. "There it is, it's right here!" she exclaims (meaning?). After two more times explaining, she goes to the barrel and dumps the bag.

Finally, we are there at the cafeteria. Servers insist on getting her responses rather than letting me order for her, which makes it difficult. I know she has preferences, but she is stymied and can't verbalize her choices. The line backs up as I struggle. With a little encouragement from me, she eats well and we leave. "You must be tired," she says to the cashier and gets her smiling, as she had done with another person earlier.

1:30 P.M. Brief visit to church offices. Jane does well and stays near me without too much jesting, and I am able to offer some direction and encouragement to the staff on an issue at hand.

2:00 P.M. Next we go to the home of a very weak, terminally ill man. Jane visits with his somewhat discouraged and tired wife, while I go to the back bedroom with him. My time is blessed, and Jane and the hostess seem to get along well, too. Though we are only five minutes from our home, Jane questions over and again whether we are headed right.

As I get our things from the car, she goes for the mail. This time I'll be sure to see what she does with it. The problem of mail retrieval is of great concern to me, but so far I can't think of a solution.

From time to time I can hear her walking near my study door and expressing aloud her concern about where I am and what I'm doing, without directly intruding.

3:30 P.M. Just dawns on me, I failed to line up cleaning service. Procedure is complicated. Cleaners must not show until Jane is out.

I want to go to the fitness center so am trying to prepare her for giving me up for that hour. This is getting more difficult now.

I hear her say to herself, "Well, . . . I don't think I'm doing very well . . . but I think I'm doing better than you might think" (trying to keep up her courage for another day).

I always call back from the fitness center after a few minutes. When I check in today, she actually remembers to tell me that a phone call has come in for me. It is exciting to me; she even tells me the name of the one who called—a frequent caller. When I arrive home, she comes into the garage to meet me, "I was beginning to worry—about to cry. No, I was okay."

5:00 P.M. Now, I try to figure what to eat. We were so hungry at noon that my original plan of having doggie bags from that meal for tonight evaporated when we ate everything. But I don't want to eat out again, so will need to get our meal before changing my sweaty clothes.

I go to the refrigerator, and again God answers and opens the Red Sea. We end up with meat and a canned vegetable and a potato that I halved between us, plus ice cream.

Little challenges at every turn in the meal preparation as I try to involve Jane without getting into difficulties. Example: "Please take the silverware to the table. No, I mean put it where we usually sit. No, not the corn; put that pan back and take the silverware. Here, I'll help. This is your plate. I'll use mine in the microwave with the meat."

After eating, I help steer dishes into hot water and redo what is necessary, and then the phone rings, which excites her. "Hurry, hurry! You'll miss it!" Each sales call must be explained as to why I did not prolong the conversation.

7:30 P.M. I receive a serious phone report of a marriage breakup from a friend wanting to help the couple. Jane goes to bed on her own. I manage to get her up and into the bath, promising to help her bathe. I try to do this at least three times a week to give hygienic support to her efforts. She now needs help getting out of the tub. We have fun together, and she goes to bed happily—partly clothed with day wear, as usual. Here, I do the best I can at holding to normalcy, but I always lose when I confront her on some issues. (Besides, I love her.) I do manage this time to get her to not wear hose to bed, noting carefully which pair it is so I can get them in the wash.

10:00 P.M. Bedtime, and I just remember that I have not finished in the kitchen. I manage to keep up on dishes and other things there. Jane appears in her bathrobe to say, "I love you; I really love you." (It's easy these days to stay in love.)

Next, I recall tonight is time for trash barrels to go out, so I make a final roundup of all baskets and some of the "attractive" plastic stuff I have tucked away, out of Jane's notice, and get everything out. As I return, I find her in the garage peering out after me.

I invite her to come out back with me to see the moon—and get a nice moonlight kiss.

Finally, I'm going to get my long-delayed bath from working out hours ago.

11:30 P.M. I note the time; Jane is fast asleep. Often she begins to speak of bed before the evening meal. I point out that the sun is still up, but it seems to her a foolish reason for not going to bed.

It is the same with eating. No sooner had we entered our home from our meal at the cafeteria than she was asking, "When will we be getting something ready to eat?" Stopping her eating between meals is difficult because she is so often in a state of neutral — waiting for a lady to come, waiting for me to finish something, waiting for the next meal or bedtime. She no longer really reads, though she sometimes goes through the motions. The piano is all that is left for her.

The coming of any repairman means I must be at home. For example, I was in my study when one repairman asked her, "How many children do you have?" She answered, "My husband . . . he knows." I helped the startled man understand.

So far I haven't been able to propose any hobby or craft that fits her in this present state. For example, all the new linen flowers and craft materials I bought for creating arrangements lie scattered about the house with other "collectables," in disarray.

I try various methods to have her share in prayer and Scripture with me. Her prayers, always so strong and robust over the years, have all but dissolved. At meal each day I have her pray at least once. Often, she quietly waits for me to pray. "No, you pray," I then say. Whereupon she looks puzzled and picks up her fork. "Please, thank God for the food! Will you do that?" "Yes, but I have to fix this first," pointing to something. We both bow again, and after a period of silence I look up and she is staring quizzically at me, waiting for instructions. We begin over again and sometimes succeed, or I pray instead.

Having full devotions together (even brief ones) is a larger challenge. For example: "Jane, you read first." (I'm hoping for a few words by her.) Long period of silence. "Will you read?" "Yes, I will." "Okay." More silence. "Are you at the right place?" Scripture references are no longer meaningful, so I must show her again. "See, right there." Then we begin again with silence. I think she is reading, but she can't get the order to her vocal equipment to

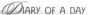

make the reading aloud. Then, prayer won't work. Since she can't remember what I just suggested to pray about, not even one thing, she invariably goes to her ingrained habit of praying right from the open Bible. Only problem with that approach is that she can no longer recall how to do it and simply resorts to talking aloud about snatches and phrases she sees from any text that her eyes happen to light on.

I have no idea how all this will appear to the few of you to whom this is directed, but I have a strong yearning for someone besides me to look in on all that I am into and to share feedback and perspectives with me. I don't think I'm mistaken in feeling that God is truly supporting and helping me, but at times there is an awful sense of aloneness.

Obviously, this diary contains only highlights of one day. Another consideration: the diary represents one of the more quiet days. Jane had my attention the entire day and was spared many of the demands that agitate and trigger angry outbursts.

Even before mailing this diary account, it is already outdated. Significant changes have taken place. For example, morning delusions or hallucinations are now bringing agitation toward me and involve wild stories. At this point, she still comes back to reality and makes every effort to reach out to me, often asking forgiveness. All of this hurts a lot.

I have always considered Jane to be a very unusual woman, so I'm not surprised that her Alzheimer's case seems to be unusual also. Here is one very typical episode these days.

Sunday afternoon, the day before the diary record, I took Jane with me on an emergency call to the hospital. I stopped at the restroom. Then, returning toward the place where my wife was waiting, I heard a man with unclear speech pouring out his heart to Jane, across the entire reception area, where they sat opposite each other. She also was replying.

As we walked away, I asked, "Did you understand what he was saying?" She replied that she understood none of it and added, "Maybe he was drunk." She felt he needed to talk, that was all. He was touched, I could tell, and he apparently did not need "right" words from her.

Such experiences come at a time when she can recall almost no one's name, not even her own sons' and daughters', but she continues a kind of spontaneous ministry wherever we go, if there is an opportunity.

Please give me your impressions, and if you help me in this way, this very time-consuming recording will have been worth the effort. I beg you, pray for us. Thank you, and God bless you.

Inside a Broken Mind

"You are kooky! Look at you!"
—JANE, TAUNTING HER REFLECTION
IN THE MIRROR

A MAN IN PERSONAL CRISIS CAME TO OUR HOME TO SEE ME. HE HAD BEEN released recently from prison and felt he was seriously failing to live as a new Christian. Jane answered the door and began to entertain him, much to my delight, while I got myself ready. Soon she was singing a very touching song about God's willingness to forgive one who stumbles and falls in life. (This occurred while she was still able to sing and play a bit.)

That God had apparently guided my wife to sing right into the man's heart the very message he so sorely needed made an impression on our caller. Later I thanked Jane and explained how important a thing she had done. Her response was simply, "That's why I chose that song." A thrill went through my whole being: This was the very person I'd always known!

DOES JANE REALIZE SHE HAS ALZHEIMER'S?

People who love Jane and are concerned for her well-being usually get around to the question of whether she comprehends her own situation. Probably that is the question most frequently asked me by those who know Jane. The answer is complex.

Let me show how it is. I say to her, "Come here to the bathroom."

"What?"

"Come right here to the bathroom."

"I don't know what you are saying."

Because Jane's hearing is perfectly normal, it is clear that she does not understand. Furthermore, she knows that she does not understand. But she does not understand that she does not know. She cannot process crucial data to the point of understanding, but she is definitely aware that her mind is somehow failing her at this point. Mercifully, though she knows there is a problem, she does not understand its full significance.

A New Kind of Language

Regardless, daily conversation has come to depend on learning a new kind of language — one that has kept changing day by day. Some exchanges are easy; others, more difficult or impossible.

Here are some of Jane's simpler challenges: "Please tell me what you are telling me" (which means, I don't understand your explanation). "Where is . . . where is you?" (I was looking for you; now I see you). "Daddy, I'm so glad . . . I . . . you" (I'm so glad I have you).

Much communication is more difficult to understand. "You know what? You are longer than you ought gotta not be" (You know what? Your face is extra red). Jane was looking intently into my face when she said this; I had been rushing about and had just sat down again to my bowl of hot soup.

"Where did the man, the boy, go?" I answered by asking Jane, "Do you mean our new dog?" She asked back, "Our *dan?*

What *dan?*" Later she pluralized the notion: "I hope our children will be happy with each other." In this way she comforted herself by imagining that the dog was not alone in the yard.

FROM PAIN TO PAIN

Like the efforts of wounded prey striving to crawl out of their brokenness, some expressions issued from Jane's own pain as surely as they caused pain in others. "I want to be a *real* person." "I'm not bad, am I?" "Am I doing something wrong?" "I'm just a little kid."

While still able to write, and standing at the checkout counter with pen in hand, she pled, "Honey, what is my name?"

Jane once was taunting her reflection in the mirror, as Alzheimer's patients are prone to do. "You are kooky! Look at you!" Then she added, in a kind of concession, "Your hair is pretty." It is not always possible to tell which role she is assuming in these debates and arguments; this time, she had recently been to the hairdresser.

I'M THE ONE WHO DOESN'T UNDERSTAND

My hope in purchasing a selected prize dog was that he would prove to be a diversion for both Jane and me. One day, however, after months of intense effort on my part, Titan decided to break all the training rules. Pondering my exhaustion and frustration, I entered our rear door looking like I felt. Then Jane approached me and spoke tenderly, "Dad, you are making me feel sick."

"Do you mean I am looking angry because of the dog?"

Jane nodded and I promptly apologized and sought divine help to better bear my burden.

Once, as we were leaving the home of friends, Jane helped herself to a hard candy (as she feels free to do, even in stores!).

In a moment or two we were seated in our car, and she handed me the empty wrapper. Seeing no trace of its contents, I asked where the hard candy was. She indicated no understanding of what my inquiry meant. When I persisted, her answer was delivered with a definite philosophic air, "They say people can do anything they want. That is what I did." After driving and thinking a while, I realized she was telling me to give her personal space without questioning her every move. The candy ball went unfound, but I discovered a new insight.

LEARNING, LITTLE BY LITTLE

The person Jane always was, she still is, at least in certain ways. Not all is yet destroyed, and I feel that the tiniest residuals are so precious they ought to be cupped in hand as long as possible. For example, she is a most observant person. While being led to the bathroom at a predawn hour, she is noticing everything along the way—where the dog is, or why some item is out of place. However, her real glory is in studying the skies. Over and over again she exhorts me to look up at the stars, moon, clouds, birds—whatever is up there, anyplace in nature. Only the dull and the doomed will fail to notice these wonders, she warns me.

Again, Jane has ever been sensitive and proper in demeanor. Alzheimer's is merely pushing this characteristic to the extreme when she lashes out with a rebuke to any loud person who visits us or sits near our restaurant table. Also, having lived more than seventy years as a highly resourceful person, she is quick to set straight one who dares address her in a patronizing manner.

One road bump that a bit of insight smoothed out was in the area of ordinary communication. I might say to Jane, "This is your place," as I pointed out which was her dinner setting. Often in response she would motion to it and say, "This is your place." One day, it dawned on me that she was not correcting me so much as merely quoting me.

Careful, thoughtful listening made Jane's heart windows more accessible. "Boy! You look good, Harold." Then, with lowered voice, "I wish I did!" Here the real person struggles against Alzheimer's battering, and it challenges the caregiver to support the wilting sense of personal value. Once, as we embraced, she whispered with perfect clarity, "Be especially close to me today, won't you?"

SEARCHING FOR THE BEST APPROACHES

Nothing is as futile and counterproductive as trying to get a slow-moving dementia patient to quicken the pace. Life is simple, with but two options. Work well ahead of schedule, or have no schedule. "Let's walk just a little faster," used to be my frequent exhortation, until I came to realize that her limbs were already moving at the top speed allowed by her confused brain.

A large test for me has been to keep trying different approaches, realizing all the while that most tactics will not work, and those that appear to be effective will fizzle all too soon. For example, I used to pit the reasonableness of my request against the unreasonableness of her refusal. I might even buttress this approach with an appeal for her cooperation with my loving efforts in caregiving. So many noble words down the drain! Besides, such elaborate efforts can build nothing for the future. All is forgotten at once.

"No! No! No! You take care of yourself!" is what meets my striving to get Jane dressed. Finally, I take her advice and go into the bathroom to shave. Directly, she comes to the door.

"Do you want to get dressed?" I ask.

"Yes, I want to be a good person." No repentance here, only that Jane wants to be a "prepared" person, ready for the day.

Next, I begin the process of relocating each article of clothing that she has confiscated from my neat stack at the foot of the bed. The bra she has carefully folded and placed beneath a napkin on the table; stockings are in her robe's pocket, and other pieces are here and there. Then we begin again.

"No! No!" From the vocal tone and body language, I figure this to be a true refusal, so I leave again. This response in turn brings a protest from her that I interpret to mean, "I want to get dressed, and you are no help." This contradictory misfiring of the brain shuts me up to but two alternatives: (1) leave her alone or (2) try again to lead her out of her confusion.

Incidentally, my repeated, patient attempts worked, and I saw it more clearly than ever: the path to winning is indeed narrowed down to simply yielding, and yielding yet again.

LOOKING DEEPER YET

Especially in dealing with hallucinations, this principle of yielding must be clung to. Invariably, my dementia charge will commit all her resources in battling any reasoning concerned with these more extreme irrationalities. Sometimes I am drawn, almost driven, to demonstrate how a particularly disruptive delusion is without basis in reality. Her best response might be to up the voltage in her presentation. At worst, a rift is declared between us. "See, even you reject me and don't believe what I say!"

Never is a single inch gained by my rational arguments. It's always downhill until I choose the higher road. Such stubbornness on Jane's part has nothing to do with any event in real history, only with Alzheimer's. My task is only to affirm my love to her and overlook this symptom of the disease.

Interesting but pathetic are my partner's struggles to appear rational, to enter into conversation, and above all to enjoy some of the recognition that she perceives is now lost. "I'm not a kook, you know" and "I can think, too" were often heard in months gone by.

Ministering to these pleas for inner support frequently required interrupting projects of mine that were crying out to be completed. "Come with me; I've got to talk with you. I need to show you something." On arrival at the designated spot, I might hear an embarrassed "I forgot." Or Jane would fumble about to produce a substitute item and line of thought to go along with the just-hatched fantasy.

THE NEED FOR RECOGNITION

Jane accosted me one Sunday after I came down from the pulpit with, "You didn't even look at me during the sermon!" She made the same complaint once in my study at home. Placing herself behind me, she said, "You don't even look at me!" She was referring to the lack of eye contact and to my often-abrupt answers to her.

Personal recognition is a key issue for most of us, but maybe even more so for one whose most precious faculties are being lost. This issue became clear when I began noticing that whenever a companion took Jane out for an hour or two, an angry outburst nearly always occurred within a minute or two after their return, even before the kind lady had left.

Finally, I saw the obvious. Behind the flurry of Jane's repeated rings of the doorbell and thumps on the door was an enthusiasm at being reunited with me. After greeting Jane, however, I turned naturally to the guest to inquire how things had gone with the two of them and to express gratitude for the help. Meanwhile (if only I had been sensitive enough to see it!), my wife felt she was being ignored. "You never listen to me!" she might blurt out. In time I realized that she was really saying, "You are not noticing me. I have been away from you for what seems like a long, long time, but now I'm here. I love you and want your loving attention."

THE PAIN OF BEING LEFT OUT

A more difficult dawning came to me while we were guests of another couple. Repeatedly, Jane interrupted our conversation with rather insulting blasts at our host. "Please don't," I begged. "Let's have a happy visit."

"Well, can't I say something?"

Suddenly, like a needed revelation, it came through to me. Although Jane's approach was not appropriate, her intent was only to contribute to the chatter. I then realized that this behavior was because Alzheimer's had destroyed her judgment as to the bounds of propriety long before speech and the desire to socialize had been lost. To her, it seemed that everyone was talking on and on without her participation. I had to confess, that was true.

Furthermore, the pace and vocabulary of ordinary conversation far outstripped her capacities to receive with understanding. "I can't hear you!" she would despair, meaning that she could not understand what was being said around her.

Left out of conversation too long one evening, Jane burst into things with, "I want to say something, too!" This announcement silenced us all, while she took center stage with a few moments of uninterrupted, pitiful, meaningless sounds. Then, knowing she had successfully intruded, even though she couldn't make herself intelligible, she settled back on the couch smiling.

Few who hosted us knew how to involve Jane in conversation. In social situations it increasingly became my task to ask Jane questions, refer something in the discussions to her, or remind her of connections with our past. As the disease progressed, this challenge became increasingly difficult for me as well, so friends are certainly not to be blamed for their inability to involve Jane.

"ANYONE HOME?"

Outside my closed bathroom door I heard a plaintive, pitiful little cry, "Anybody here? Anyone home?" Somehow, that soft call shook loose a thick layer covering my understanding. I saw it quite plainly for the first time. The reason Jane intruded every few minutes (or even seconds!) wherever I was in the house was due to her memory loss. Once out of sight, I was really lost to her.

With brow furrowed and eyes moist and reddened, Jane burst into the house from her three hours out with a companion. "I thought I had lost you! I was afraid . . . afraid you'd be gone before I got back." Encumbered with diminished capacities to evaluate all the data reaching her fouled-up brain, Jane is nonetheless a person whose sufferings must not be ignored. I see her as a beloved, struggling soul lost on trackless seas where rage many a storm. Some of her painful anxieties I can fathom and help; many more she bears with none sharing. At least, this exasperating situation brings about many healing hugs that warm my heart, and I believe hers also.

SURPRISE! I'M STILL HERE

As startling as an unexpected bolt of lightning were those passing moments when Jane's brain suddenly "worked" again. "Be careful of that!" she warned, pointing to my wallet, about to fall from the table's edge.

Within weeks of that experience, we were sitting together on the den sofa. I muttered to myself, "I cannot recall what today's date is."

"Why don't you look there," she said, pointing to the daily newspaper. Unable even to say "newspaper," she somehow, for that moment, knew how to help me. Then the ability was gone as quickly as it came.

DEEP WITHIN HER BROKEN MIND

Until recent days, Jane and I discussed her disease, with some understanding on her part. I wanted to keep abreast of how things were deep within her heart. Each conversation flashed to me the same two signals: (1) the gravity of it all did not grip or much concern her, and (2) her main interest was in seeing evidences of tender care on my part. The following conversation, often duplicated, always led to the same encouraging conclusion.

I would ask Jane earnestly, "Does this problem with the Alzheimer's disease trouble you? Please tell me."

"I don't really think about it."

"Remember, I love you, no matter what."

"That's all that matters, because I love you so much! Just don't ever leave me. I don't know what I would do. . . . "

"Honey, God is helping me to love you more and more, and I won't ever leave you. Do you believe I love you with all my heart?"

"I know" (with tears). "I know you do."

Her devoted love makes my task easier. During all the typical Alzheimer's angry outbursts, I try to keep in mind what I know is deep within her heart, as distinguished from what the disease foments for the moment. It ain't easy! But God helps one to do whatever he commands.

4

Love That Lives
Through the Fire

"I am so glad God gave you to me, and I love you with all my heart."
—JANE, WHILE STROKING MY FOREHEAD AS I
AWAKENED FROM A BRIEF DAYTIME NAP

WHAT KIND OF LOVE CAN COEXIST WITH ALZHEIMER'S DISEASE? IN THE previous chapter we glimpsed some of the tangled thinking that has overgrown Jane's mind. Here we look at the love that is able to live in such a thicket of thorns.

No amount of fun and encouragement itself can be the cause of love that is real and that lasts. Rather, such love is capable of generating good humor, creative effort, and a determined faithfulness to help sustain itself.

One is born to lifelong agony whose feelings are quickly aroused by needs of others but whose will to act is lazy and without discipline. I suppose we have all met people like that, who go through life gasping and groaning—forever retching but never reaching.

I try to keep these things in mind as I relate to Jane. Sympathy must not outstrip the will to act. Alas, I must confess that at times I am barely hanging on.

45

If love were only visceral, no caregiver could love his or her ailing spouse. Alzheimer's is a disease that makes a relentless assault on the patient's physical charms, emotional well-being, intellectual capacities, and bodily mobility. Alzheimer's destroys the *person*. All avenues of expressing personhood are steadily shut down.

One spouse is losing the other. And the ill one is losing enjoyment's grasp on every earthly thing. Both caregiver and patient are Alzheimer's victims.

COMBAT OF THE UNCONQUERABLES

The love of which I speak is a committed relationship that springs from the will of one person toward another. The accompanying outflow of affection and sacrifice might or might not receive a rewarding return, but the response will not stop love. It extracts its strength from the veins of opposition.

Scripture says, "Many waters cannot quench love; rivers cannot wash it away" (Song of Songs 8:7). Love's flame is inextinguishable. Alzheimer's, however, does all in its power to snuff it.

What happens when these two invincibles deadlock in battle? The disease gradually tightens its hold on the beloved patient, and the caregiver is staggered. The one most loved becomes in so many instances the most repelling! For hours at a time, the flow of love is only one way, from the tending one to the one being tended. Not a word of gratitude, a tidbit of sympathy, or a morsel of mercy reaches the beleaguered caregiver from the spouse. At best there is an utter unresponsiveness; at worst, abuse.

As the cruel monster is finishing its prey, the victim's stubborn, negative resistance is silenced. Then all responsiveness is stilled. Companionship ends.

The only kind of love that still stands, after all this, is that which is by choice. It is willing to pay any price to meet the need of the one loved. I frequently ask myself, What would I want Jane to do for me if I were the one in need?

Thankfully, at this writing, Jane is still responsive to some of my efforts. She might, for example, pronounce over my head her benediction of grateful love as I am kneeling to ease her aching feet. Or she may look searchingly into my eyes with an expression that I would describe as a mixture of anxiety, longing, and trust. My heart responds to this. Were it not for my love, she would be left to the ravages of fear, because I am her only contact with the world of reality as it slowly slips from her.

"My mind doesn't work; I am losing . . . " she once tried to explain to me in a very special conversation. I then and there promised again, "Jane, I will be your mind. God will help me, and I won't ever leave you."

"I know, and I love you so much." With that, she nestled her face against my chest and seemed content and happy once more. Those conversations are now largely in the past, but the memory of them often energizes my sinking heart.

Here and there, expressions of devotion still burst forth, such as, "I thank God he gave you me!" I know what she is trying to say, but even taken literally, I like it. I like it even when she calls me "sweaty" (for "sweetie").

ALZHEIMER'S KNOCKOUT PUNCHES TO THE CAREGIVER

Multiplied inner conflicts arise and reside somewhere in the pit of one's stomach. The advance of the disease makes it more difficult to be with my partner and at the same time more difficult to be away from her. There are times when emotions are all spent, and at least for that moment, the last person on earth I wish to see is my beloved. In marches the prosecuting attorney of the conscience, and I fall in an anguish of guilty feelings before the trial can begin.

Too much introspection is destructive. Love is proved by what it does, not by what it feels. On many occasions, I must do what is right by choice, against how I feel at the moment.

In great need one day, I came across a verse in the Bible that gives a simple two-step plan for getting through the swamp of discouragement. Here is now my regular companion: "So then, those who suffer according to God's will should commit themselves to their faithful Creator and continue to do good" (1 Peter 4:19).

This Scripture instructs me to (1) commit myself to God and (2) put one foot in front of the other and keep on doing what is right. Inevitably the clouds part, and sunlight again comes.

Many and varied are the piercing arrows flashing from Alzheimer's and finding their mark in the vulnerable caregiver. Here are several examples, as typical as they are painful.

Jane once stared blankly at the TV, ignoring my repeated questions. I was trying to get from her some hint as to where she had placed a carton I had seen her carrying about. "You're not answering me; what are you doing? What I mean is, why are you not answering me?"

"I didn't want to get blasted." Her answer jolted me. Flurries of questions rushed through my mind. Was I being harsh? Or were her feelings only the accumulative result of day-by-day corrections and restraints that are so "necessary" to assist any dementia patient?

Near the top of the list of concerns is the matter of time and attention. Losing all ability to concentrate on any constructive or recreational diversion, the patient becomes pitifully dependent on the primary caregiver. Time spent separated from me seems indeterminably long and even threatening to Jane, no matter who makes what effort to divert her.

Many a time, on returning home, Jane has burst through the front door, leaving behind the one who had taken her out for a time, calling urgently, "Where have you been?!"

"I've been right here working until you came back."

Then her deeper feelings come out as I am holding her, "I thought I had lost you!"

Another time when I had been pressing to get work done in spite of her many interruptions, I became aware that Jane had not been around for a while. I finally found her in the family room, looking lonely and dejected. Kissing her and holding her tight, I winced at what she said: "I didn't think you wanted me anymore." At once I reassured her of my love, and I also silently cried out to God to help me remember how things appear to her.

Life with a dementia patient is life with a *real* person. Patients are persons; it's that simple. ("Simple," though, does not mean easy!)

Laughing one afternoon at my cheer-her-up antics, Jane said, "Oh, this is fun! You know, I don't get much time."

"You mean, with me?" Very solemnly she nodded yes, with head tilted and eyes searching deep into mine, making sure that I got the point.

Long before the severity of Alzheimer's advanced phase, each new experience brought the pain of things to come. Less than a year after the diagnosis was given, Jane phoned me at the church to say that she could not figure out why suds were overflowing from the washing machine. "You need me to come home, don't you?" I said.

"Yes; I'm so sorry!" Arriving home, I found her looking pitiful and defeated. In my arms, she whispered, choking, "I'm so sorry I'm ruining your life." At that, I fell apart and just sobbed on her shoulder. No matter how hard I struggled to remember that I was there to support her, I could not stop weeping and gain control.

Perhaps all turned out well, because she needed to be needed.

During this phase, a friend would sometimes take her shopping. From one such trip Jane returned triumphantly holding out to me a purchase made especially for me—more aspirin-type tablets. "But we have tons of this stuff already!" I said, demonstrating my early ineptness at caregiving and my insensitivity.

At once, I was taught my lesson—indeed, it was branded into my heart. My dear wife turned sadly away and pined, "If only I could go to heaven and make right decisions and not do foolish things."

Valentine's Day was close upon us, and I purchased four cards and gave them to Jane over the next several days. In response, she bought me two at once, writing in them very touching words. I was dumbfounded that she could still write such words. They were her last written words of love to me.

Later that week she mentioned her sadness at losing her memory. Various related losses were cited. I pointed to the quiet but strong influence for good she still was in our church. "I need you to help me," she said. "I can't find any book in the Bible now. All the truths and lessons I taught are gone from me."

"I know, but I'm your memory, and we'll make out together." As the months passed, such conversations ceased, but they were painfully precious while they lasted. Once, while she was detailing, with clarity, her distress at the disappearance of faculty after faculty, she noticed mist in my eyes. "You starting to cry? It's my turn, you know."

JANE'S PRESENT LOVE FOR ME

There is no question but that love between a devoted husband and wife can become more deep and profound even while Alzheimer's teeth continue to devour.

There are two ingredients to this love. The first is Jane's love for me. She never comments directly on the sacrifices that I make in caring for her. She might, instead, resist me strongly. Even so, I have learned that service lovingly rendered seems to layer-in a foundation for positive relationship. And eventually,

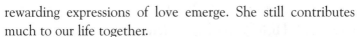

rewarding expressions of love emerge. She still contributes much to our life together.

A case in point might be trying to shop with her. We had neither bread nor milk one day, so I insisted on her cooperation with the inevitable. It was a difficult time. Back at home, I had an hour's worth of tasks to do in my home office. Getting her to allow that time was another contest.

A few minutes later, she was back with a clearly stated apology, "Sorry if I make it hard for you."

"No, Jane, perhaps it is I who needs to repent." With that she withdrew, only to return a moment later with reddened eyes.

"Why is it I love you so much I just want to cry?" she asked.

Another evening while intensely involved in a study project, I became aware of her presence in the doorway. Softly and with great deference she spoke. "I won't bother you; just want to be near, where I can see you."

To me, it is almost miraculous that amid all her loss and humiliations she still has hours of genuine joy. "Oh, I have never been so happy in all my life!" is a frequent exclamation. These expressions are like flashes of the last light of her life, and they reach my heart with a reviving force. I know that all too soon these final glimmerings will darken permanently.

Jane's own comforting acts and words touch me more deeply as I realize she is reaching out to me from her heart, without understanding what our situation is all about. Sometimes when we are in quiet enjoyment of one another's company and her mind is functioning better, I return to the question, "Does your sickness with Alzheimer's trouble you?"

The last time I asked her that question brought this clear, succinct reply, "No, you will help me, won't you?" Everything within me rises up with desire to be faithful to such a trust.

While preparing for bed one evening, Jane brightened things up by calling out, perhaps to me, or maybe addressed to

God in praise, "It is so wonderful that God gives us people to love us so!" I believe this had reference to my tending her during bathing and toileting. Often she thanks me earnestly at each step in the processes.

More than once she has touched my forehead with tender concern, exclaiming, "You are hot! Please don't be sick. I need you so much!"

When my wife breaks free of the disease's agitation, she showers me with compliments. They are said with such earnestness that I am always taken by surprise. Once I awakened from a brief daytime nap as she was stroking my forehead and whispering, "You are God's man. I am so glad God gave you to me, and I love you with all my heart." (There's a moment worth dying for!)

My Love for Jane

Besides Jane's love for me, a second ingredient needs added focus: my love for her. Only two alternatives are left to me — duck out of the relationship, or love her and serve her. I do not resign myself to the hard task of serving her. I willingly choose it because I love her. Before I explain how this love originates and continues, let me highlight it yet more.

Her needs, as I view them, are of two kinds: those that attract sympathetic response and those that strongly repel. As an example of the former, imagine how I felt when she, grieving over her failing ability to play the piano (which she has done since childhood), said, "I can't play the piano as I used to . . . it's my head."

Feelings of love easily welled within me. I ached for her as I held her and sought to console her. "Please don't grieve. We'll get through."

"It's okay as long as you love me." Any husband's love would tend to rise up at that. Mine did.

It was a far different story when at 2:00 A.M. urine flowed out on the edge of the bed. Her outcry was not soon enough, or I did not awaken quickly enough. She was upset, the bed and the carpet were being soiled, and I was unprepared for all that was yet to happen.

To Jane's broken, agitated mind, my insistence on moving her directly to the toilet area, removing the dripping nightie, and washing her made me a main part of her perceived problem. With all her might she resisted me, battling and blasting her way back toward the carpet. I stopped her, declaring firmly, "Jane, please don't. I'm stronger than you, and I can't let you leave until we have finished."

Still holding her firmly with one hand, I bowed to pick up the soiled clothing while she rained blows on my back and head. "I thought you were my husband!" she cried.

Within minutes she was again quiet, and I was able to restore her inner balance and kiss away the turmoil. As I was changing my own clothing, Jane asked with genuine, tender concern, "Anything more I can do to help you?"

"No, I guess I'm all set now; thanks for everything." Then back to bed for two spent people.

The Secret Source of Love That Lasts

As I have already illustrated, dementia hits the attending partner with a wide range of challenges. When the very one you love the most says, with deep anxiety in her eyes, "I don't know who I am anymore," love mounts on wings of sympathy, at the very least. It is the same when, in discouragement, Jane asks me to hold her, and studying my eyes and facial expression, she pleads, "Honey, don't ever leave me!"

Coming up with appropriate, sincere words at such moments is not all there is to love, however. Love must be gotten before it can be given.

I believe I know the secret. "God is love. Whoever lives in love lives in God, and God in him" (1 John 4:16). God has set himself to help us if we come for help. Putting it plainly, we need our needs. Desperate situations must not separate us from our salvation's source but, rather, drive us to it.

But that is only the front half of the matter. After the input of God's love, there is the day-after-day test of giving out love, even when intensely frustrated or pulverized by grinding routines. Because I love, I can, without support of natural emotions, make the difficult, right choices. I can choose to avoid an argumentative tone or harsh attitude, which communicate more readily than words, to the one suffering from Alzheimer's disease.

Instead of surrendering to each tough scenario, I must keep telling God, myself, and Jane of my love for her. Rather than allowing each futile attempt at conversation to dangle from another dead end, why not use it as an opportunity to interject an "I love you"? Additional love flows into a caregiver's heart only if there is a commensurate outflow. Being unable to remember even minutes earlier, Jane never thinks it extreme or redundant if I stay at it all day, each day. Love thus grows.

During the period of this writing, I was tucking my wife in bed one night and saw in her eyes that the last light was brighter at that very moment. Quickly, I began a meaningful discussion with, "God has given us many good years of life together and of ministry to others."

"Yes, *many!*" she said emphatically.

"I love you, Jane, for all you have done for me and for so many others."

Her eyes filled with tears of recollection and acknowledgment. I held her tightly, trying to cling to that precious flash of understanding. That light left, but love stayed.

5

Withering Experiences

"Get out of here with your sweet talk!"
—JANE, FEELING THAT I WAS BEING
CONDESCENDING TO HER

WHAT IS THERE ABOUT ALZHEIMER'S DISEASE THAT TURNS THE CAREGIVER'S mind to pulp? First, if the patient is a spouse, then that caregiver is losing his or her dearest loved one in a painful, protracted burial by increments. As Jane loses her mind, I lose my wife, bit by bit, faculty by faculty.

Second, the one you most love will often hurt and even attack you, verbally and physically.

Third, the more the patient needs correction, the more resistive to it he or she becomes.

Fourth, if you commit to in-home care, you thus commit yourself to a lock-in with one suffering from dementia. Your own emotional and mental perspectives will surely come under fierce siege. Patience will be pulverized, tender feelings bruised to the point of bleeding, and all resources drained. In brief, your life will seem to be chained to the task of trying to figure out how to do what you cannot possibly do.

Here are snapshots of personal experiences that tended to wither my spirit and would have broken me had not God been merciful.

NO WAY NOT TO BE WRONG

Our early days together in the dark tunnel had their special hurts. While Jane was still attempting to teach Bible study lessons to individual women, she felt trapped between her desire to continue this ministry and a growing awareness that the resources of her memory bank were diminished. She had been exceptionally gifted in this work over many years. As far as I dared, I encouraged her to continue on a limited basis. Alternately, she would discontinue her meetings with one and consider engaging another. When I sought to caution her ever so gently by reminding her of how difficult it was becoming for her (and, no doubt, how troubling for others), all her pent-up frustrations poured out.

"You are cruel! You don't know how hard I try and how much I want to do this. I am not copping out. I've served you well over all these years!"

Naturally, I did that which was exactly wrong. I attempted to allay the hurt by explaining what I meant. I had yet to learn that explanations are very wearing to one suffering from Alzheimer's. The downward spiral continued.

"You are nice to others but not to me."

"Please tell me what you would like to do. Do you wish to continue teaching? If so, I will try to help you."

"Get out of here with your sweet talk!" And then searching through her arsenal for a weapon with more clout, she came up with, "People will one day find you out for what you are!"

Rays of understanding at last began breaking through the clouds. I saw that Alzheimer's always holds the caregiver to choices between undesirables. One simply must bite this bullet and stop looking for escapes. And it is far better to bite the bullet before it is fired! That is, don't be backed into decisions. Hard, undesirable courses of action are not necessarily wrong in the eyes of God.

When I first came to the realization that Jane's problem was some form of dementia, I longed to share this burden with the family, the church, or anybody who would listen. However, I felt bound by the notion that her rights and also our vows of love and loyalty would be breached. It seemed to me, in my early perspective, that the moment I disclosed our secret, very large and irreversible changes would take place regarding her ministry and mothering. She would forever after be viewed in a different manner, I reasoned. As time passed, however, I learned how futile it was to delay coming into the light with our plight. Getting the whole matter into the open enabled our love to flourish, with support from those who understood and cared.

Furthermore, back then it was a nightmare hearing her say things that were incorrect or inappropriate without making valiant effort to correct them and keep her in touch with reality. I felt complicity if I did not keep trying. But that way not only didn't work, it did harm.

NO MORE MUSIC

Song left our home, and silence crept in. As one by one Jane forgot how to play her various instruments, she would set them aside without comment, exactly in the reverse order in which she took them up. First to go was the organ. Next was the autoharp, then the vibraphone. Finally the piano, played from childhood, has slipped from grasp.

Music had been a part of my childhood also, and Jane and I became acquainted singing together on a daily radio program in Boston. Our children sang and played instruments. The loss of music in our marriage was crushing to me. I tried various methods to encourage her to play as I listened or to sing again with me, or even to play as I sang. But what Alzheimer's takes, it doesn't give back. Tears and pleading cannot change that. What is gone is gone. Continuing to adjust to the inevitable is the only recourse.

LAST COMMUNION

Sunday, July 2, 2000, was a day I will remember, for that was the first time Jane balked at taking communion. I rescued the bread from her toying fingers and ate it along with mine. Next, I whispered to her the meaning of the cup, but it did not register at all. Sadly, I passed her by with the tray. Now that understanding has so failed, I judge that this will have been her final communion.

SHOPPING KEEPS YOU HOPPING

Entering a supermarket with Jane was at times like stepping into an arena full of wild animals. With dangers looming and lurching at me on all sides, my task was to calmly fill my cart with desirables and empty it of my partner's contribution of undesirables. Worse yet, she felt free to help herself to fistfuls of goodies from any open display. I would rush to each crime scene and faithfully proclaim to unhearing ears the inappropriateness of that behavior.

All mirrors and reflective glass along the way had to be adroitly avoided, or I could expect an explosion of arguments with her adversary—her reflection. People within hearing distance could only suppose that I was her object of wrath.

Then there was the trail of puzzled shoppers whom Jane felt she must cheer up as we moved along through the store. Even if they desired to be thus greeted, her choice of words must have mystified them. I could not come up with a standard assist to the situation, so it usually was left dangling.

In each store, every several moments, I heard, "Let's go home. I want to get out of here!" This response taught me how

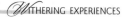

she must have felt when, in earlier years, I was impatient on shopping days.

PUNCHING OUR HOST

On another occasion, we went to some friends' home for dinner. "Get out of here!" Jane ordered the host, just as we entered the house.

"I live here," he said with a smile, and then dodged a hard punch thrown by his guest. My pleading, "Let's have a happy evening, please, please," had little impact.

In our own home, what feelings of helplessness paralyzed me when a guest was told, "You're fat!" or "What a nose you've got!" (Try as I might, I've never thought of a way to uninsult a victim.)

My hope was that this very uncharacteristic anger would prove to be but a phase in Jane's disease. Time has indeed moderated it to some extent. Some of the worst outbursts, though, are reserved for me, with ample supply also for friends she sees most often.

These shoving and punching attacks did not usually hurt me physically. A few times I tried warning her, "I am bigger than you; I am not at all intimidated by you, and if you don't simmer down, I might have to paddle you." It doesn't seem very nice to say that, and I have never done it, but I keep hoping to see a warning work. Not so far.

The only option remaining to me was to keep telling myself that she in no way was aware of her wrathful outbursts. As time passed, all became nothing more than a grueling routine without the painful edge.

FROM ALL SIDES (VARIETY IN MISERY)

I quit longing for the experience of sitting down to one of my wife's prepared meals. Gladly would I have settled for being allowed to prepare the meal myself in peace, without the table being unset as soon as I had set it, without having to settle some emergency with Jane, or without having to convince my dear partner to come back again to the table.

On another note, the disappearance of so many of our friends was somewhat surprising, even though I had been fore-warned to expect this development. I was sure they simply weren't comfortable with an Alzheimer's couple, so I was not deeply distressed over it. All the same, the long and tedious hours made me appreciate an evening in another home and also made me thankful for faithful ones who did not forget us.

Periodically, I sat myself down and tried to prepare for days ahead when there would be less motion and sound from Jane. I knew that some patients become very unresponsive. Meanwhile, we walked ahead together amid ceaseless barrages of repetitious verbal expressions, such as, "How are you? What's going on? Huh? Huh?" (repeated up to a dozen times, or until I answered.)

Again, I might ask her, "Did you have a good sleep last night?"

"Who?"

"You."

"For what?"

Then she might ask, "Why do you say it that way?" (prob-ably meaning, Why are you inquiring?). To end this cycle of monotony, I had to respond with a vague answer.

I never discovered an effective method for checking on her meanings. Often, when I tried to resolve things with, "I'm not sure what you mean," she would reply cheerfully, "I don't either!"

DENTURES ON THE DINNER TABLE

For reasons known only to an Alzheimer's mind, Jane removed her lower denture and refused to put it back or allow me to do

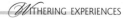

so. My repeated efforts to remedy the situation caused us to be late for a dinner appointment. We walked into our friends' home—she with dental plate in hand. Casually Jane placed it on the dinner table in front of her place setting for all to see.

WALKING ON GLASS

A miracle! That is how it seemed to me the morning that Jane plowed right through the middle of a sea of broken glass covering the dinette floor. Not one piece pierced her bare feet.

It all began with a crash and our guilty dog hurrying into the hallway from the kitchen to escape my scrutiny. The picture, then, was this: The dog was on one side of the glassy sea (finely shattered remains of a large, fragile drinking glass), and I was there attempting to erect the expandable barrier to hold him in the rear hallway away from the glass. But Jane arrived at that very moment and was about to stroll across the sea, despite my shouts to the contrary. At once, I abandoned efforts to block the dog and rushed with the barrier back to the other side of the glass (crunching it under my shoes) to restrain my wife. Calling to the dog to stay, I also warned Jane of the danger. Making the mistake of thinking that she now understood and would cooperate, I dashed back—with barrier still in hand and glass still underfoot—to our excited young German shepherd pup. I quickly slammed the barrier into its place, only to discover Jane standing behind me. She had walked through, barefoot!

The worst struggle, however, was just beginning. When I attempted to keep her at bay while I cleaned up the glass, she became incensed and literally fought me, trying to walk again from the kitchen into the dinette—and through the glass. Each time I released my hold on her arms to deal with the glass, she stepped into the danger area. The situation was desperate. Finally, I grabbed a table chair and pressed her down into it. "Please don't make me have to hurt you," I begged. I don't know what I meant by that. But I felt the need to say something strong and shocking, and that was all I could come up with at the moment. It didn't work. Nothing did.

After what seemed like a very long time, she simply gave up the physical exertion and relied on verbal abuse. Sensing the change, I cleared up the glass in record time, finishing up by brushing gingerly over the area with moist paper towels. Then a thoroughly spent, very thankful, and utterly amazed husband examined the unmarked soles of his wife's feet, and life returned to the Alzheimer's normal.

TWO PATIENTS IN THE HOUSE

How impossible everything still seems anytime I became ill! A desperateness develops when I am unable to attend to my own needs, let alone Jane's. Once when my head was not just spinning but swirling violently, I was unable to sit up or even move my head at all. Ultimately I was taken by ambulance to hospital emergency care. My wife became excited and perplexed.

"Stop looking like that!" she shouted. (But how does one make the green go away?)

Then she tried pounding me on the back while ordering loudly, "Stop acting that way!" No way could I figure how to convince her it was no act but the real thing. Moments later she was pleading, "Don't be sick. If I lose you, what will happen?" Whatever heart I had left went out to her, but until help arrived, our situation seemed very black.

TOUGHEST OF ALL—THE GRANDDADDY OF ALL MY GRAPPLINGS

The toughest struggles, however, are with Jane's incontinence, especially if the accident occurs when I am not well. A combination of these two trials plunged me into what proved to be

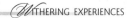

the darkest, most furious combat to date.

Before recounting it, I must explain with thankfulness that Jane is not fully incontinent at this time and generally sleeps well, nor has wandering away from home become a major problem. Those major Alzheimer's problems have spared us to a certain extent so far, but the dementia is not thereby disarmed, as I will now show.

I was set up for the disastrous episode by spraining my ankle chasing our German shepherd around and around in our enclosed back yard. Instead of teaching him a firm lesson, I fell flat on my back in pain — only to receive comfort from the miscreant himself, as he stretched out inside my arm with his head cradled on my shoulder, quietly waiting for me to gather my senses. This was another hospital emergency, with the verdict being "severe sprain; keep off your feet as much as possible; use crutches."

How does one on crutches give a bath to an uncooperative person? The answer is, in pain. A long night followed my first attempt, while hobbled, to bathe Jane. But I was not yet fully ripe for Alzheimer's knockout punch. The next day, my effort to recoup lost sleep with an afternoon nap was cut short by Jane's repeated efforts to rouse me. I counted some fourteen of these none-too-gentle intrusions. Finally, I arose to face the remainder of the daylight hours, tottering about on the crutches and not suspecting the big event near at hand.

I will let a letter to our family tell the story. After describing my deteriorating injury, I chronicled that next, fateful night:

> Just as I was getting pretty helpless, if not worse, everything fell apart in the predawn hours. Jane urinated over the mattress and across the carpet (while I was pulling her and yelling all the way to the bathroom). By then she was so excited and confused that she refused to be seated and completed the matter in a large pool on the

bathroom tile and mat. Then she fought like a tiger as I attempted to remove her soaked robe. Finally I left her there, went out to the middle of the room, and cried good and loud.

Then I went back to her as she attempted to bring the problem out on the carpet. With great force, I stripped her and battled until I had her somewhat washed at the sink. (I knew I had not enough strength left to bathe her fully. The physical struggling and working on hands and knees hurt my sprain.) Surveying our "battle zone" and considering the continuing struggle with a very upset AD person while hopping on one leg, I decided to phone for help. Hated to do it at that hour, but . . .

While I was on the phone, I heard another outcry from Jane, and lo! she had loosed a postscript on the carpet leading to the other bathroom and over that tile and mats. There she stood with another nightie soaked and in need of more washing herself. I could see immediately that this nightie would not go over her head without soiling her hair, so I pled with her to let me get her arms out so I could drop it to the floor. World War III (or was it IV?) resulted. I tore it off her with great physical exertion and threw it into the main pool. Then I got her washed, dried, and into the guest bed.

Meanwhile, Titan had gotten the drift that he would be executed on the spot if he intruded. He went to the far side of the guestroom bed and stayed there quiet, even when our friends arrived to help. Another couple of hours and we were done, at daylight.

Today, I am worse in my fat foot with its toes sticking out from the swelling and beginning to discolor. Mary Ann spent the entire day purchasing a new bedding set (which was needed anyhow), feeding us supper, and both of them returned tonight to finish up things. Now they have gone,

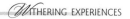

and I am about to seek to bathe Jane, etc.

I need to tell you something more. I was awakened this morning an hour before all this happened, so I got to the bathroom for myself, or there would have been another big problem. But more important than that, as I awakened, the Spirit spoke graciously to me the hymn,

> Be still, my soul! The Lord is on thy side;
> > Bear patiently the cross of grief or pain;
> Leave to thy God to order and provide;
> > In every change he faithful will remain.
> Be still, my soul! Thy best, thy heavenly Friend
> > Thro' thorny ways leads to a joyful end.

Wonderfully, in the midst of the nightmare at its worst, that message came back to me, and I was sustained. So I love the Lord, for he has heard my cry.

Amen, by his grace,

Dad

A Reprieve

A little occurrence that I cherish happened amid all the yelling and striving at its worst. My hair had fallen across my forehead, and Jane for a quick moment suddenly stopped fighting, gently brushed it back—and then promptly resumed the war. Jane is for me, not against me; this I know.

Each day following the incontinence, however, the insistent questions about my crutches continued, "What are you doing?" "What is wrong with you?" Nothing was remembered about her accident or why I was hobbling about. Appeals to her for a more sympathetic cooperation were virtually ineffective.

REFLECTIONS ON MY WITHERING

I suppose that every Alzheimer's caregiver is initially mistaken about what to expect. Does anyone know how far down "down" is, until one gets there? Each time a record low is hit, the darkening thought looms, How can I possibly handle those worse things that are yet to be? As for my present "withering," I cannot say that I feel green and flourishing, but I have, with God's help, withstood some of the shriveling exercises.

Humor — and Lots of It

"Oh, Daddy, you are the best I've seen in years . . . about two years."

—JANE, WITH A TWINKLE IN HER EYE

EVEN LITTLE LIGHTS ARE BRIGHT WHEN THE TUNNEL IS VERY DARK. HUMOR often provides a respite for Jane and me from the thickening shadows of Alzheimer's. Sometimes funny things just happen, popping into the routine like a burst of sunlight. Other times, I contrive them.

Very early in our life together, Jane and I both realized there was quite a difference in our two propensities to comedy. From the Boston area, she is much more reserved and reticent than I. Her marriage to this Southerner required daily patience with his pranks and his efforts to liven up the home for our four children.

For example, I once came up with the idea of a mystery ride that would fit our very limited budget. The children were each given a large paper bag to place over their head once they had gotten in the car. It took extra effort to "bag" my wife, but she finally agreed "for the children's sake." Finally, I drove out of the driveway with my five brown-bagged riders (one still mumbling a bit). The journey was underway! With many comments designed to keep them confused, I proceeded to a mall parking lot close by where I could mimic stopping at traffic lights. After turning in various directions, I left the lot and proceeded to our destination—a nearby ice cream stand. The treat (not to mention the unbagging!) was a delight.

COMEDY IN CAREGIVING—IT HELPS

Over the years Jane's funny bone gradually thawed until she began to initiate many comic activities and sayings herself. This pattern has helped us both during the present trials. She seems to grasp humor more readily than many other kinds of exchanges.

One day Jane had me a bit bruised and reeling from her angry verbal assaults, so I asked, "But you do love me anyhow, don't you?"

"No, I don't!" was her firm answer. The tone left an opening, however, to appeal the decision. I pictured the two of us in a courtroom before judge and jury.

"The judge is about to speak," I declared solemnly. "Ladies and gentlemen of the jury, you have witnessed Jane's life with Harold. Does she truly love him? What do you say? What is your verdict?"

From the "jury" came my resounding "Yes! She does indeed love Harold!"

"See there? I knew it all the time," I added. Jane looked knowingly at me, making no admission, but obviously enjoying the fun. The tension was over.

PUBLIC BURPS AND EAGER EATING

My embarrassment over things like Jane's loud burps in restaurants gradually sank into the oblivion of overload. When guests were present, though, I felt that some response was demanded. Here was one of mine: After an incident, I asked our friends, "When an explosion that loud occurs in a nice restaurant, do you know how to tell which patrons are veterans of war combat? Just look around; they're the ones peering out from underneath their tables."

In our home one day I followed her burp with my own counterfeit. "No, not that way!" she protested, objecting to the artificiality of my effort.

To upgrade the presentation, I removed my glasses and held them vertically to serve as a monocle, announcing, "I shall show much better class now and burp with a British accent." I am still perfecting that one.

The urge to help herself to food includes anything on nearby plates during the preliminaries of a meal. By the time a prayer of thanks is finished—especially if it's a long one—even our host might have a short serving. No matter where we are, the sound of crunching food has become familiar background music to table grace.

JANE'S OWN HUMOR

My wife's particular style of fun-making was always a bit different. Now that it is debilitated by Alzheimer's disease, much of it is lost—but not all.

Some of Jane's foibles I classify as being humorous simply because they help me get through what otherwise might be an irritating moment. Recently, while trying to invent another meal, I looked back to see a large, bite-size hole in what I was preparing. Nothing is safe and secure when Jane is lurking about the food—especially if she is hungry. I admonished her sternly and continued my work, only to discover seconds later that the entire portion had disappeared along with the hole! Its replacement also met a similar fate. Finally I moved the entire operation to a safer spot.

FUNNY SAYINGS

Here are several examples of Jane's sayings that have struck me funny, some uttered to herself seemingly for her own amusement:

- "We are not there because we are here."
- "How old would I be if I weren't here?"
- "We are not as bad as we are."
- "One never knows (said philosophically) . . . I've got a nose, too" (laughter).
- "Thank you, Daddy. You are a really, really good man . . . once in a while" (said with a whimsical glance at me to see if it registered properly).
- "You are the best I've seen in years . . . about two years."
- "If you don't know what you don't know, then you won't know you're nosy."
- "Where is the honey? I thought I was your honey" (said smiling, after I had commented about the honey I had just spread on our muffins).

KABOOKA ADVICE

The approach of Sunday brings added responsibilities to a pastor's life. Jane seems to have retained some of this perspective from our half-century of ministry together. On a more recent Saturday, long after the disease had devoured most of our sensible conversation, I quipped, "Well, tomorrow is Sunday, and I've got to have a sermon. Do you know any good sermons?"

Walking away from me, she called back, "You'll have one by then. Kabooka-booka."

JANE SHOCKS EIGHT MEN

Weekly, a group of men gather for prayer at our home. On one occasion Jane decided to sit in our circle. The group showed understanding, and, I must add, my wife was quiet for the hour-long meeting.

After the hour was up and while we men were busy saying our good-byes, Jane hastened unnoticed to the front hall. As our guests turned into the hallway, they were confronted by my diminutive wife blocking the front door. With arms outstretched so as to forbid their exit, she declared with no uncertain authority, "I'll put down the first one who comes!"

A wave of shock rolled over the men. Quickly, however, it turned to cheerful laughter. Their loving respect and tact soon gained them safe passage without injury. Jane quite obviously enjoyed their reaction.

SPARKLING DIALOGUES

Harold: "You look nice this morning, Jane."

Jane: "Well, no, you look worse."

H: "Please come and finish dressing, honey. You look funny that way."

J: "I know I do, and I like it!" (spoken clearly after a morning of speaking only gibberish).

J: "Look what's coming under the door!" (spoken with startling clarity—Jane's attention was focused on our patio door, with its loosened "tail" of weather stripping).

H: "Hey, it's a snake!" (She was delighted when I joined in the joke.)

J: "Oh, honey, I don't know when I've been so happy."

J: "What are you doing?"

H: "I'm trying to think of what we can have for dinner. I'm not very good at getting meals, you know."

J: "I have nothing more to say at this time" (spoken with a witty air).

J: "I was just thinking . . . not stinking but thinking" (laughter). (These words, muttered more to herself than to me, piqued my interest and stirred hope that I might get to her mind's window while the curtains were once more slightly open.)

H: "What is it? Remember, you were saying, 'I was just thinking'?"

J: "Well, I don't know myself. I forgot." (With that, the curtains closed again as tight as ever).

FORTY-NINTH ANNIVERSARY BOOGIE

As the date of our forty-ninth wedding anniversary approached, I decided to abandon all logic and attempt an overnight trip. After all, I reasoned, there was little chance that intelligent relationship would be present for our fiftieth.

We made the trip with understanding friends who arranged reservations in a well-appointed inn at nearby Williamsburg, Virginia. Having completed a nice dinner, with a number of surprises supplied by Jane, the four of us retired to our rooms. Our friends were in a room down the hall from us.

If someone had been outside our door there in the hallway that night, that person would have heard immediately the sound of all three locks in our room being secured. And a few moments later, the same sounds again as Jane unfastens the locks. (Trouble is, I do not hear anything, for I am brushing my teeth at that precise moment.) Next, out she strolls into the hall, barefoot and wearing only her little nightie.

Sensing the quiet in our room, I soon discover the reason. Abandoning my toothbrush, I charge out of the room in my own informal attire. Too late I think of the door. It slams and locks behind me. Now there are two of us locked out.

Looking this way and that way, I see no sign of Jane. Soon I hear a faint sound in the distance. Down the hall and around the first bend, Jane is happily giving a full-voiced lecture to the corridor walls. It is a painful sight. She looks so pitiful and out of place!

Hoping no one comes upon us, I hustle Jane down the hall and back to our door. One lady does spot us, however, peering wonderingly from her doorway to see what we are up to. My only option is to persuade Jane to remain at our door while I dash for help. I rouse our nearby friends with, "I need help!" Then I hurry back to retrieve again my wandering spouse. Shortly, one of our still-understanding friends joins us in the hall, views our plight, and hastens back to his room to call the front desk.

Keeping Jane cornered at our door was growing more difficult by the moment. What has happened to our friends? Where is somebody—anybody—with a key? Reappearing, our now dressed friend informs me that the woman at the front desk cannot leave her post. "I'm going down for a key," he says.

Several minutes later after we are restored to the privacy of our own room, and without expecting any answer, I go through the motions of remonstrating with Jane, "What on earth were you doing out in the halls dressed like that?"

Looking straight into my eyes and with a grin of delight, she replies, "Boogie! Boogie!" It is very difficult to hide my amusement, but I manage as best I can.

Next morning, after we are dressed, Jane makes another brief escape into the hall, but I catch up to her just as she is shouting commands to staff workers down the hall, "What is that noise? Who is making that noise?" Not waiting for any confessions or investigations, I pull her, key in hand, back to our door.

Other unexpected events added color to the remaining hours of our getaway celebration. We arrived back at our quiet home with the question in my mind, Why did we do that? And yet, deep down, I was glad we did.

MIDNIGHT WEDDING MARCH

I was faintly aware that Jane was stirring in bed. That was the last thing I wanted. I was sick, and had already carried myself to the bathroom about ten times. Managing a half-cheerful "Here, I will help you; please get up," I hurried around to her side of the bed. The battle began.

"Come to the bathroom."

"What bathroom? Where? Where?" I reached under the cover for her feet and turned her body into a position to sit up on the bed's edge as prelude to standing. Anger ignited, but it worked nonetheless. She was soon moving.

A distance of about fifteen feet separates bed and bathroom, where the night's toughest challenge was to take place. So I made the most of our little walk by intoning, "Here we are — two lovers walking hand in hand (this physical contact is essential) down the roadway of life." Ludicrous enough, considering the setting, but nonetheless purposeful.

The contest that developed was made more insistent by the fact that I did not know at what moment her weakening capacities of bladder and bowel control would reveal themselves. Around and around we went as I tried to get her to sit down, then use the tissues, wash her hands (soap on one hand and then the other), rinse her hands ("both hands, please"), dry her hands on the towel, return to the bed, climb back in her side (not mine), and — "Slide down further so your head doesn't hit the headboard."

As tedious as all of these struggles are, I'm sure that they would have been much worse had we not had the pleasantries on the way. In spite of her broken memory, humor's residual is there, layered-in deeply by years of experience. Our fun awakens this capacity, I believe, and provides an ameliorating resource to draw on.

Even if my wife were not being eased a bit, I would still use these lighter moments to escape the tightening grip of self-pity. And for all I know, maybe down in the depths of Jane's heart, she somehow senses this value of humor and is willing to go along with it. Anyhow, we soon began practicing a new version of our bathroom march, using an exaggerated hesitation step and singing softly, "Here comes the bride. Here comes the groom. On their way to the ba-ath-room."

As tough as it is to do in the wee hours or whenever one is exhausted and not well, things would be a lot tougher without the effort and aid of humor.

For Those Who Are Caregivers

"Boogie coplocket plocket. What's a plocket?
Do you know what is a plocket? Huh? Do
you?"

— JANE, WITH SINCERE URGENCY

THE COLLEGE OF DEMENTIA CAREGIVING HAS NOT YET GRADUATED ME. MY qualifications to write this chapter are largely limited to what I have learned through a decade of dealing with a single patient, Jane. Some of my understanding and practices are without doubt uninstructed, but I hope they will be of value. Surely, commonalities exist among Alzheimer's cases. Also, I take comfort in the excellent material readily available to aid caregivers with questions on which I might not have been clear and complete.

Here then are insights presented in three categories: a short list of progressive challenges faced; identifying the true enemy; and hints for caregivers.

PROGRESSIVE CHALLENGES AWAITING THE CAREGIVER

The first category of insights involves a chronological look at the key phases or critical junctures through which I saw myself being drawn, pulled, and yanked as Jane's disease developed. Movement through the progressive stages of Alzheimer's is unpredictable, and the one attending inevitably must make countless adjustments. Learning must be welcomed. Here are key phases in caregiving as I experienced them.*

Earliest days of unrest and disturbance. Because the problem is not yet identified, no way can be found to resolve anything. Unprecedented unreasonableness on the part of one spouse is met by growing frustration and unhelpfulness on the part of the baffled partner.

Suspicion of dementia. The baffled partner likely begins to suspect dementia. The next problem is how to introduce professional assistance. First, I got Jane to agree that she was not in her best condition of health and that something was harming her memory. "Let's find out what it is and what can be done about it," I reasoned with her. A bit reluctantly, she went through the battery of psychological tests.

The diagnosis of Alzheimer's. The neurologist or the primary physician brings this dreaded conclusion to the family member who is in charge. This step forces to the forefront the issue of whether to tell the suffering one, and, if yes, when and how to

---

* A call to any local chapter of Alzheimer's Association will make available the latest and best books, tapes and videos, area support groups, upcoming conferences, and other resources a caregiver might need. It will be noticed that I have avoided the use of mood management by medication. My "tools" will be obvious to the reader—sometimes nothing more than outlasting a phase that appears impossible for a time. Caregivers, in consultation with their physician, will have to decide for themselves what medical means to employ. One aid that I have found extremely valuable is "Safe Return." An identification bracelet bearing the patient's number provides immediate linkage between the Safe Return headquarters and local, concerned persons.

do so. In my case, I took the advice of a nurse and of a doctor. The nurse encouraged me to go through with my plan to inform Jane. Then she shared this insight, "Telling her won't stop the bad times, but it will aid during the good times, since she will better understand and cooperate." The doctor proposed that he be the one to tell Jane, which was done directly.

Informing family and friends of the diagnosis. Following quickly on the heels of the diagnosis is the matter of informing family and friends. Such a disclosure will alter forever the way they view the sick loved one. Still, it must be faced that Alzheimer's cannot long be hidden. Any attempt at silence exacts its own price. As erratic behavior escalates, so do rumors. It's true that people and situations differ, but much is to be said for the direct approach of going public with the whole, correct story. Then people around can offer support, rather than contributing to the problem.

The long next phase of endless learning and adjustments, until death brings its parting. This phase might be divided into many parts. I will mention two segments of struggle that have caused me the most concern thus far. One is deciding on the level of assistance you will require and employ. Very early the question must and will be faced as to how much strength and endurance the primary caregiver has. Which of the options, for any required assistance, will be pursued? (Thus far, I have been able to keep Jane at home with me, using some volunteer help and limited professional support. Most of the hours are still mine to cover, alone.)

The first several occasions of leaving your helpless loved one in the care of a hired caregiver will be painful. For me, I struggled with feeling that I was deserting Jane, who was antagonistic toward the nurse's aid and begged me not to leave. No matter how I reasoned things, I grieved for her, much as if I were consigning her to the death of a meaningless life apart from me. In spite of all this, I recall a distinct sensation as if a pulley belt had slipped free, leaving the engine to spin without a load. It had been so many months since I had such hours of release, I was somewhat disorientated. Each conscious delight was followed by guilty feelings that I was neglecting my wife.

Fortunately, before venturing into the plan, I had made the decision that, during the days of getting used to everything, my head would rule my heart. Placing one's spouse and home in the care of an outsider is not altogether a happy happening unless the one engaged is a well-trained, efficient, and sensitive person. At-home care agencies are generally available to recommend and place workers. If needed, for an added fee, they will provide supervision.

One major concern is the loss of sleep the caregiver often suffers. Other problems can somewhat be adjusted to, but stressful nights bring a crushing weight of a new order to the caregiver's schedule. (When and if I face the full twenty-four-hour watch, I will look first at in-home nighttime options.)

The second struggle in our final long phase is dealing with incontinence. The onset of this problem will prove to be a most formidable confrontation. I crept into these days feeling like one standing at the edge of a vast wilderness of many dark, twisted experiences—all totally unfamiliar to me—and for which I was totally unprepared.

Yet, as incontinence continued its unrelenting progress, my changes in caregiving somehow kept up. If asked how I get through these days, my answer is, With many a groan.

As already indicated, I was not prepared. I should have read more, counseled more, planned more. My ignorance regarding the newer designs in absorbent undergarments increased our woes. My overriding concern was to protect Jane's pride and stay as far as possible from "diapering" her. Trying for that ideal without the aid of modern accessories put a strain on me day and night.

Here was my plight. Though I faithfully watched the clock, timed each trip to the bathroom, and awakened at any restless stirring in the night hours, accidents still occurred. For one thing, Jane's physical systems were gradually changing—from age, if not from Alzheimer's. In addition, the disease confused her mental control center that operated the containment and release of bowel and urine functions. Sitting there on the toilet, Jane simply could not always connect the urge with the relieving command from the brain. Nor could she understand my prompting words. All these factors, together with the fact that she wore no protection, made me feel like one playing Russian roulette. Each loss meant another unpleasant cleanup operation.

Very soon I discovered various undergarments that would contain the mishaps without offending my wife's pride. The stressful worry is now gone. I still time bathroom visits, but I keep a container of moist wiping cloths handy and sometimes have to give an extra bath and do emergency laundry. Zipping our bed mattress in a plastic cover and using absorbent pads make sleep easier.

IDENTIFYING AND CONQUERING THE REAL ENEMY

Spotting the elusive Chief Enemy and dragging it into the light of understanding has not been easy for me. My wife certainly is not the enemy. In fact, she is not in any way an enemy. I myself am the only possible candidate.

If I willingly accept all the burdens of an Alzheimer's caregiver, in what way might I be the foe? *By acting without adjusting.*

Alzheimer's drives one key message home to every person who tends one of its victims: This progressive sickness will end in disastrous grief unless there is substantial change, and then more changes after that. The changes are not abstractions but are real and essential. Because only two persons make up this intense relationship, it is easy to see who must face up to the responsibility for making them.

These ongoing inner adjustments allow the caregiver to act in an ever-updated manner, matching the patient's alterations in mood, behavior, and mental capacities. Once the caregiver becomes accustomed to (one could say "skilled in") making crucial adjustments, and doing so often, things will be much easier. Seeming impossibilities in coping will give way to new approaches that remain undetected until the caregiver ceases fretting and despairing and comes into a new willingness to change.

Frustrated caregivers not only fight themselves but also draw the ire and fire of their patient. That makes two against one! Fortunately, if the Chief Enemy surrenders, the other combatant will more likely follow suit.

SOMETHING TO SETTLE ONCE AND FOR ALL

When the full weight of homemaking and caregiving ultimately descended on me, I was stunned by all the difficulties. Even the physical challenge was far beyond what I expected. Life became a hopeless thrashing about in the dark—hopeless, that is, until I agreed with the inevitable.

One day I took solace in this line of reasoning: Alzheimer's puts every caregiver in over his or her head, so it's not so important that I do not stand as tall in abilities as some. Still, I had to face up to two inevitables. First, my assignment is plain hard work and will get increasingly more difficult day by day. Second, it takes all day, every day.

False hopes are folly. Two phantom notions drift into my thinking regularly. One is the forward look toward some positive change and better days. Another inviting, but harmful, idea is to plan outside projects that I wish to accomplish in addition to the household duties and caring for Jane. These side glances of desire only breed discontent and frustration. If other tasks must be done, or if time for recreation is required, arrangements should be made for assistance in rendering the basic tasks.

In my case, I found everything complicated beyond measure at the outset. The microwave mystified me, and skills in handling women's apparel eluded me. (My full confession, I think, would encourage the most disheartened caregiver!) Homemaking is becoming easier. As for the caregiving, I am finally feeling more natural at it, though the demands keep changing and intensifying.

THE SECRET SOCIETY OF THE SORROWFUL

Membership among those who silently grieve is not optional. You must and will join. Even though you might for a time find willing ears to hear your woes, very soon you will drive them away. They will feel they already understand, and you've told them repeatedly. Of course they do not really understand unless they are married to a dementia patient, and of course you have new, painful experiences yet to tell. Only one course is open to you. Talk at length to the one or two who might invite it, and learn to weep alone in God's presence without despairing. Jesus is a fellow member of your society of suffering.

Once quieted and less distressed, you will be positioned to take new, practical steps of improvement. Perhaps you can benefit from the ideas I present under the next heading. There are ways around, or through, many seeming impossibilities. Keep in mind that the darkest of tunnels is a way through an impossibly high mountain. Contrast your tunnel with a cave. In the latter, the further in you go, the further from the light you are. Not so with your tunnel. Keep going straight ahead, and you will break through into the light again. That experience will then be behind you and will give you confidence for the next foreboding mountain ahead.

There is no way around, or over, the full range of trials, so my advice is, Cease striving for what cannot be, enter the tunnel of the required. Keep performing the next-due responsibility. In time, each tunnel will be traversed. That is how it is to love and care for one with Alzheimer's.

Hints That Might Help

The following list of forty hints and examples is certainly not exhaustive. Perhaps, though, it will trigger thoughts that go beyond the immediate suggestions.

Keeping Positive — and Realistic

1. Don't panic at any impossibility. Working consistently and effectively in the uncharted havoc associated with Alzheimer's is truly a skill. No amount of expertise, however, can get an unwilling person in or out of the bathtub or can remove dentures through clenched jaws. Avoid exasperation, let time pass, and make a fresh approach.

2. Develop the art of "surfing." Don't fight the waves of emotions. Use them. I am no paragon of patience, but this concept has been of immense help to me. A surfer does not shake his fist at the ocean when it fails to deliver the wave he wants. No, he waits and waits for the big one. If perchance some contrary force dashes him under, he still does not rage but rises and waits again. Catching the wave must be learned by experience. Practice "reading" the patient's moods and notice what might contribute to brighter emotions. Use the highs to accomplish the more difficult caregiving routines.

Examples: For Jane and me, it is best to set bath time in early evening before weariness and negative feelings set in. I create a pleasant atmosphere and then ride the wave. In dental care, overnight soaking of dentures gave rise to great problems. Mornings are down times for Jane, until after breakfast, but dentures are needed before breakfast. Solution: Clean the plates well at night, soaking them during bath, and return them to her while she is in good spirits after bath or as I am tucking her into bed. (Ultimately, for us, this issue resolved itself when Jane decisively rejected further use of dentures — which led to a new set of problems.)

3. Don't worry about tomorrow's problems. Many a dark future will brighten when experience brings new insight. Nothing stays the same; changes occur in the patient, in the situation — and in the caregiver. Remembering this helps to combat despair as you consider what is ahead.

4. Stay clear about what your main task is. When there is a conflict between a project of the moment and a duty to your loved one, ask very carefully, Which is the interruption, and which is the main work? Never view the suffering one as standing between you and all the things you want to do, whether work or recreation. Forever settle it: the patient and his or her needs are your grand objective. If you are anything like me, this issue will require a determined, once-and-for-all decision that is renewed day by day.

Example: As I once hurried by Jane on my way to accomplish a task, she called me to look with her at a carved wall plaque, as we had done many, many times in the past. Following a leisurely look and appropriate comments, she burst out with, "Dad, I'm so glad you are good with me!" Not only was I rewarded, but also I was reminded of something crucial. Deep within, Jane is evaluating my responses to her. It's in my power either to lift her up or to let her down.

5. Bring a clean slate to each difficult caregiving assignment. If you encounter confusion and agitation *and* what sounds like a final refusal to cooperate, try standing quietly aside until things settle down. Then make a new approach. If that does not work, quietly walk away and return later. If that fails, take time to create a change in atmosphere. Express your love. Refer to pleasant memories of the past. Use momentum: "Let's get the bath done as quickly as we can; I want to sit in bed with you and read."

Example: A lady who came to take Jane for a ride had difficulty getting her into the car. Presently, my wife headed back toward our front door with the companion following helplessly behind. Back to the car the three of us went. Jane also refused my attempt to get her into the car. Rather than reasoning with Jane or taking her arm and pressing her to step into the vehicle, I simply stood there behind her, saying nothing. Then I retried with quiet confidence, as if it were the very first effort. This time Jane responded positively. She was acting in reference to the immediate context, not to the previous struggle.

6. Hold on in patience and persistence through each difficult period. For example, stages of very angry resistance and hallucinations ultimately pass into other phases that may be more manageable.

7. Expect some positives. Take heart, some things will get easier as your own tastes and tolerances change—but always you must practice accepting the unacceptable.

8. Recognize and accept the irregular as routine. Look at all unchangeable behavior—no matter how grating and time-consuming it is—as nothing more than a routine responsibility in your assignment. Dealing with unreasonable irregularities is what it's all about!

9. Expect behavior below ability. It is not enough to determine what the patient can do unassisted. Increasingly, things the patient can do, he or she won't do.

Example: I lay out Jane's bathrobe and slippers on the foot of the bed so that when she awakens each morning she can slip them on and not be cold. Invariably, though, she carries them about until I help her put them on. Often she steadfastly refuses to put them on (especially the slippers) until after breakfast.

10. Expect the patient's phobia-like fears to replace rationality in certain areas. I think of the fears as fill-ins where there has been brain loss. At any rate, unwearying initiative is called for.

Example: Jane's dread of having her nails cut pitched her into panic at the sight of the clippers. I didn't heed her pleading so she upped the voltage with intense physical resistance. I gained a temporary reprieve by taking her to a podiatrist for a problem with an ingrown toenail. Watching how he made the cut and purchasing similar clippers helped for a time. However, she continued the practice of jerking her hand away from me. Then I came upon this technique. I sit next to Jane but at an angle with my back toward her, wrap her arm around my waist, and trim her nails away from her sight. That seems to work. Other solutions might be to try it while the patient is asleep, or to trim a nail or two each day.

11. Plan how to deal with "walking" objects. If the patient begins to carry around, relocate, or lose things of value, devise a plan for their systematic collection, sorting, and disposal. As painful as this solution might be, neglect will prove more painful.

12. Keep thinking and thinking about possible solutions. If none can be discovered for a particular problem, see if you can devise a way to outflank the difficulty so it won't have to be faced head-on.

COMMUNICATING WITH THE PATIENT

13. Make wise daily preparations for future loss of communication skills. Establish consistent patterns in activities, caregiving, and speech. Fasten into your loved one's mind simple, essential words, supported by hand signals such as pointing, and attach them to the daily routines of personal care. Then when the patient no longer chooses to do necessary routines, your words of direction will still be effective for an extended time. Next, when even your simplest words no longer carry meaning, your hand signals will extend the period of easier care. This advice applies to each aspect of toileting, dental care, dressing, eating, getting in and out of the car, and other activities that are regularly done. Choose wisely and practice faithfully these communication aids. You will be glad you did.

14. Remember that, in communication, more is being received than is shown. Processing inwardly continues long after most rational output has ceased.

Example: Jane once showed no recognition of an illness that I was trying to hide from her. Later, however, a friend discovered that Jane was worried about me and had expressed her concern in several of her own words.

15. Resist the natural tendency to withdraw from eye contact with the Alzheimer's patient. Although it might seem distasteful at times, looking your partner in the eye is beneficial to you both. These ill ones already feel insignificant and set aside, without having their caregivers seem to discount their very presence by not so much as looking into their face.

16. Don't reply to every word spoken, but don't ignore every word. It is unnecessary—and would be maddening—to respond to each of the daily barrage of questions and comments, but it is unkind to ignore all of them. I use three grounds for determining when to answer: (1) value in the question; (2) Jane's need for recognition or interaction; and (3) opportunity for lightheartedness.

Example: Jane once said urgently to me, "Boogie coplocket plocket. What's a plocket? Do you know what is a plocket? Huh? Do you?" I leave unanswered this kind of babble question, except for occasional fun.

17. Be realistic about apologies. Whenever sensitive caregivers must make apologies, they will always feel left in a deficit position. The sense of failure may be strong, but the comprehension and forgiveness from the loved one will be weak or nonexistent.

18. Especially when leaving and returning to your patient, express your love directly. Before and especially after times of separation, make sustained eye contact and express your loving attention, regardless of who else is present. Your arrival triggers excitement that ought not be ignored or squelched.

19. Strive for balance in responding to requests. Many will be the questions, meaningless efforts at conversation, and calls for attention. Don't feel the duty to respond to everything.

Example: Jane's frequent "emergency" calls of "Come quick!" usually do not mean much, except that she is feeling anxious at the moment, although sometimes she has found an insect or might be signaling a toilet need. For peace of mind— hers and mine—I usually respond to these cries.

HANDLING THE PATIENT'S RESISTANCE

20. During heated sessions of resistance and rage, quietly reaffirm your love and assurance. Do so more often than you reissue the appeal for cooperation in the matter at hand. Keep confident in love's approach to caregiving. Even though benefits are not readily seen, love impacts the course of the disease in many ways.

21. Fight only the battles that matter. Practice the art of ignoring the inconsequential. In a tough tug-of-war, evaluate the situation, asking, Is it really worth the toll? If you are not sure, delay by deciding not to decide for the moment.

22. Remember that pleading and cajoling are counterproductive. They only stir negative reactions. Caregivers must daily recite the axiom, "As my emotions mount, so will my patient's; agitation guarantees a negative response." Then make the pledge, "I will not play into the hands of Alzheimer's." (Of course all of us will fail this over and again, but at least these principles will explain the resulting chaos.)

23. Avoid making direct challenges to your patient.

Example: Jane insisted on getting into bed fully clothed. Foolishly, I laid down the challenge, "I'll come to bed when you agree to change into your nightie." It took until dawn until I learned my lesson and I was willing to negotiate a settlement.

24. In conflict, don't just follow your feelings. Usually the way to gain cooperation lies upstream against your feelings. That means doing what you don't want to do in order to get the patient to do what you do want.

25. Choose words carefully in order to smooth the way to compliance. "Let me have that," even if padded with "please," is needlessly agitating. Avoid any reference to "taking away" things; rather, emphasize that you appreciate them and will be responsible for them.

Example: When Jane refuses to allow me to remove a piece of clothing, I promise, "I'll hang this up for you so it will be ready for next time." Every time we go outside, Jane must first relinquish her armload of "treasures." A positive approach I use is, "These are very nice; I'll keep them safe right here until you return."

MOVEMENT AND EXERCISE

26. Talk and walk very slowly. All caregivers know they should do this, but the point needs reiteration. It is not that patients won't keep up; they can't.

27. Use an open palm, not force, for guidance. An open palm placed firmly in the center of the back is more effective, when leading or lifting a patient, than pulling the arms. Also it does not seem to stir anger as readily as grasping the limbs.

28. Have the patient begin a routine of exercise early in the course of the disease. This exercise might be nothing more than a daily walk or kicking a beach ball back and forth. Stretching exercises are beneficial also. Don't surrender to thoughts of the futility of it. Maintaining a general vigor in health will give the brain support to keep functioning as long and as well as possible.

29. Plan for your own exercise and recreation. Stay with it. I work out regularly, and not many days go by but what I thank God that I am able to keep fit. Caregiving means lots of bending, kneeling, and lifting that otherwise would injure or wear me down.

DRESSING AND EATING

30. Avoid clothing that is hard to put on and pull off, anything with too many buttons or snaps. Choose simple and loose styling—anything that won't complicate bathroom proceedings.

31. Give creative thought to the patient's diet. Among the causes of nutritional deficiency in Alzheimer's patients are loss of appetite and a disorganized approach to eating.

Examples: Fresh greens are often neglected, so I serve the salad first, keeping better-liked foods out of sight. The same with fish and certain vegetables; I feature them while the appetite is keenest. Also, turn the dinner plate so as to promote things most nutritious and encourage their notice—with a few bites already cut and one on the fork. Avoid nagging. Similar thought is required for water consumption. Your strategy should include early morning, before breakfast, and between meals, as well as during mealtimes. "Please finish your water so I can wash the glass" has been effective many times.

32. Expect changes in preferences. Dislike for certain articles of clothing or food items might be only temporary. In some cases it might be a mental block or an emotional vendetta against the thing in question.

Example: A food that Jane previously relished but came to reject I withheld for a time and then reintroduced as if nothing had changed. Now she again delights in it. Recently, she gladly wore a nice sweater blouse that was for a time steadfastly rejected. Rather than disposing of it, I waited until all debate about it was over and forgotten and then tried again.

WITH OTHER PEOPLE

33. Whenever possible, prepare others for interacting with your patient. If the Alzheimer's sufferer still recalls faces, encourage friends to give their names slowly and clearly and perhaps mention a key experience or relationship once shared with the patient. See that the patient is involved in at least some of the discussions by use of questions or personal references.

34. Limit your talking about the patient in his or her presence. Also take the responsibility to direct others to do the same.

35. Do not easily give in to the patient's anxious refusals to socialize. Interaction with others is beneficial to both caregiver and patient.

SHOWING EMPATHY

36. Value the patient's well-being more than getting tasks done efficiently. Protect personal significance by helping the patient to help you. Take the position that you are assisting the patient. Keep it that way as long as possible, even though it will be more time-consuming.

Example: If modesty is an issue for the patient you are helping to dress, carefully follow the routine and order of putting on and taking off clothing that is most comfortable for the patient. In addition, I encourage Jane to participate in small ways. I pull the stockings up to the ankle, tap her leg, and encourage her to finish putting them on. Stick to the routine each time.

37. Be attentive to body language, facial expressions, and other evidences that characteristically accompany physical distresses. Do so while the patient is still communicative. Consult with your doctor as necessary, but plan and practice for the future so that you can offer input to the physician.

Example: While my beloved patient was still able to verbalize what she was experiencing, I verified the value of certain practical remedies for relieving her frequent bouts of stomach cramps. A full glass of hot water, rubbing and patting, and a hot water bottle often brought relief. Knowing how to relieve this problem might spare me having to commit to a medicine at a time when I am not sure what the complaint is.

38. Try to think how complicated everything is for a diseased mind. Insight gained in this way can make empathy easier.

Example: Notice all the steps involved in washing the hands. 1. Go to the basin. 2. Turn on the water. 3. Pick up the soap. 4. Rub the soap on both hands. 5. Return the soap to its dish. 6. Rinse the soap from both hands. 7. Turn off the water. 8. Get the towel. 9. Dry both hands. 10. Return the towel.

39. Rule out any thought of "punishing" your patient, no matter how difficult and unreasonable actions become. Blame and accountability are not involved, and failing memory nullifies the benefit of all training in the past. It will seem at times to even the most patient caregiver that the loved one is surely doing things contrived to torment, out of a kind of spite. I believe that to be both true and false. True, in that there is intent in it. But false, in that the intent is not rooted in responsible calculation.

40. Stand back and look at yourself with your patient. When that loved one is irritating you and making you angry, is not he or she only acting out the disease? Who, then, is being irrational?

What Have I Learned from the Agony?

"The person who gave this to me . . . I don't know."

— JANE, CARRYING HER DIAMOND ENGAGE-
MENT RING CASUALLY ABOUT

MANY OF THE TOUGHEST COURSES IN THE COLLEGE OF DEMENTIA Caregiving are required of all who study there. I find myself, though, pressed into a double major. Far beyond training in domestics, the School of the Spirit has tended to dominate my studies.

These transformational courses tend to be painfully personal. However, good reader, because you have come this far with me, may I share these intimate things with you? Heretofore, I have not opened some of these doors even to family or closest friends.

Much that is about to follow is fresh to me and unrehearsed in the ears of others, but I hope it will be no premature presentation of green truth. I do, however, confess to writing the preponderance of notes for this chapter just as the shades were going up on new insights. Lessons already familiar have also come to me with a new, life-changing energy. Often there were

tears—of pain or praise or both. Surely, the battle has benefited me. Trials tenderize the heart.

As you can understand, the way to these truths has not
been a pleasant avenue. Indeed, the route is worse than unat-
tractive—it is downright repulsive. But gnarled trees that
dominate a landscape, when backed by a sunset, make a pho-
tograph worth having. So, good friend, take camera in hand
and come with me a few more steps.

You see, all along I have felt strangely certain that I am on
a journey, even while shut up in our small home. Far from the
busy life I once led, I am underway to a place I much want to
be, though taking a route I dread. Just as withering plant life is
but a step removed from death and new growth, so my withering has led to enrichment. Like a death that brings new life.

One Sunday afternoon I was on my knees hurrying to get
Jane dressed in time for a speaking assignment I had, and things
were not going well. I was feeling slightly nauseated, to begin
with. One leg of her panty hose, which I managed to pull on
partially, proved to be hopelessly tangled with the other. At this
moment the phone rang. Still on my knees, I reached the phone
with one hand and answered, holding fast with the other hand
to the hose. Precious progress in dressing was quickly lost as
Jane twisted about, tying up both legs with the stocking.

Here were the results: Jane was thrashing mad at her condition. My caller, with his own problem to deal with, was wondering what I meant by, "Please, keep your leg still!" And I,
already distressed with nausea, now had a thoroughly whacked
equilibrium.

Such experiences have stirred me to ask, "All this is doing
something within me, but *what is it?*" In this chapter and the
next, I summarize the answers I have received. I try to take the
full measure of the painful situation engulfing Jane and me in
order to answer the question, When tragedy is terminal, can
there be triumph?

"ANYBODY OUT THERE KNOW HOW IT HURTS?"

With tears welling in her eyes, Jane pleaded, "Don't ever leave me. Be close. Sit by me, please!" We were in a restaurant booth facing one another. I slipped from my seat and moved in beside her. With my left arm around her, I used my right hand to feed her. We were a sight to behold.

Recent days had brought marked deterioration in Jane's emotional stability and, with that, new heartache to me. I distinctly recall, as I led Jane from that restaurant, having the urge to stand in the middle of the parking lot and shout, "Anybody out there know how it hurts?"

I sometimes consider all the miseries Alzheimer's has brought into our lives and try to choose which is the worst. Not being able to talk over anything is bad but not the worst. Christmas, New Year's, the turning of the century and millennium passed without a trace of understanding from my wife. Multitudes of other agonizing episodes have taken their toll— but none hurt so much as those moments when she clings to me and pleads, "Please, Daddy, where are you? Don't leave me. I want to be with you. Oh, thank you! I thought you didn't want me anymore." During those moments of fearful anxiety, she never weeps alone.

It dawns on me now that Jane's life has become like one locked in a prison; I have pitched my tent out in the prison yard to be as near as possible. Visiting-time allows some contact, but only briefly, and it follows no regular schedule. For the most part, I can only observe through barred and shaded windows as she wastes away locked from me.

Another aching adjustment forced itself on me when I noticed Jane had removed her diamond engagement ring and was carrying it casually about. At my remonstration, she said with furrowed brow, "The person who gave this to me . . . I don't know. . . . "

I protested, "I gave this to you for our engagement and marriage!" She responded with flat disinterest, "No you didn't."

I could arouse no recollection of our promise and vows. So, only months before our fiftieth wedding anniversary, I rescued the ring and put it in a desk drawer—for what? For forever.

ANOTHER SIDE TO THE PAIN

Consider how safe is my position. It is humbling, yes. But when one is not up, there is never a falling down. And is there not safety on the knees in prayer? Few fall off their knees.

Still fewer fall from their cross. This thought brings me to the point of this chapter and a major thrust of the book. Jesus said, "If anyone would come after me, he must deny himself and take up his cross daily and follow me" (Luke 9:23). A cross is much more than a weight to carry; it is an instrument of death. The victim is nailed fast to it.

Notice further that Jesus is saying to each disciple, The lot in life I have given you will include your own personal cross and a daily crucifying. This means an every-day surrender and a painful putting to death of selfish desires. It is hard to choose the denying of wants. A cross hurts.

I have come to realize that all these tough episodes I've been sharing are nothing other than the nails that hold me to my cross. But there is a good part, for two priceless results have emerged. First, this cross has forever changed my life in positive ways—I am a different person, not what or who I was. Second, the resulting tears have brought clearer sight. Almost everything appears different when looked upon from a cross.

WHAT I'VE LEARNED HANGING HERE ON MY CROSS

Many of the lessons that have come while on this cross have taught me how to live in new ways within my world, which—at least outwardly—is only shrinking and deteriorating, constantly.

FINDING SATISFACTION IN THE OBNOXIOUS

In the old days, a farmer might clip a chicken's wings until she learned to stay where she belonged—that is, in the pen he had fenced off for her. Likewise I had to learn that my flapping was futile and only led to more falling.

Settling down in my providential pen brought me finally to sense a strange (for me!) kind of satisfaction when I look at housework all done: the kitchen in order and without dirty dishes or crumbs, the table clear and clean, the trash out, the laundry just finishing and soon to be folded and put away. Whatever would Jane think if she could evaluate all this? More deeply yet, I wonder how God views it.

Multitudes of responsibilities concerning Jane reach out to me. On one occasion, just after a friend had taken her for an outing, I sat alone in the house thinking. I wondered how it would be with me if I were in Jane's position of extreme dependency. Next came the question: Am I doing my best—for example, when I dress her? Through the years, she always kept herself looking nice.

"Lord, help me to do the job as I ought for Jane and for you," I prayed, kneeling by our bed. As I prayed, a question intruded into my mind. When I see Jane beyond the grave and our eyes meet, will I be ashamed for having taken any needless shortcuts with her hygiene and dress?

LEARNING TO LET OTHERS LIFT

According to Job, "A despairing man should have the devotion of his friends" (Job 6:14). The one who takes on caregiving for an Alzheimer's patient will soon come to the same conclusion. Isolation is devastating. The apostle Paul begged his friends to pray for him. I do the same.

The faithful friends at church who serve as Elijah's ravens by bringing hot meals to our door three times weekly help me not only with relief from cooking. They also help me learn to receive support from others. That can be a difficult lesson to learn.

GOING BY GOD'S CLOCK

I am often tempted to self-destruct in worry while God's help is on the way. I don't always sense his enabling grace percolating in my soul. Rather, dark anticipations many times overshadow all else. Jesus spoke about the danger of borrowing our worries from what we see ahead. I am learning to notice that, at this moment, I'm still on my feet — or at least I'm alive, even if on my back. Then I commit the next upsetting scenario to the Lord in prayer, determining to wait for, and expect, his help. When relief seems late, I inevitably find that my watch is again running ahead of the divine clock.

SEEING WHO IS WITH ME IN THE BOX

God never shuts a child of his in any box of suffering unless he enters it also. Thus no matter what is shut out by the painful confinement, more is within that box than without. The trusting soul is gaining far more than he or she is losing.

This line of thought has sustained me more than once while pinched in agonizing frustration. I'm learning to think as did the apostle Paul, who saw his position as "having nothing, and yet possessing everything" (2 Corinthians 6:10). Then he wrote, "And God is able to make all grace abound to you, so that in all things at all times, having all that you need, you will abound in every good work" (2 Corinthians 9:8).

ACCEPTING THE PRUNING KNIFE

Sometimes when I take the dreary inventory of Alzheimer's toll over the days, months, and years, I feel I am cut off from God. But reading John 15 assures me that the Gardener is not cutting me off. He is cutting me back. God's purpose is not to get rid of me but to get fruit from me.

In my case, some heavy pruning has been necessary in order for me to learn to give continually without view of repayment or reward. It has meant coming up with loving reassurance every time Jane's brown eyes look toward me in anxiety, whether I am busy or not, tired or not.

And, behold, a God-given discovery is made! My giving relieves the immediate distress. The transforming benefit strengthens me, refilling my own cup, as it were. Beyond that, Jane is benefited in many ways.

After much careful observation, I have come to feel that the healthy spouse's loving investment in the ailing spouse touches and, for a time, enlivens chords once stilled by the disease. I cannot hold back the tide, but I can gain relief from some of the relentless waves. Only the "pruned" person is strong enough for this production.

SEEING SIGNIFICANCE IN SMALLNESS

A closely related point is the need to distinguish between smallness and insignificance. Sometimes, while doing dishes or some disagreeable cleanup task, the thought will come to me of the far-flung exploits of my friends. I hear of their work at home and abroad in the very ministries in which I once served, studied, wrote, and taught. Age is nibbling (gobbling!) away at me. It appears that tending my Alzheimer's wife is life's homestretch for me, and nobody is in the bleachers to see it. I hope that I am somewhat sanctified, yet I cannot help hearing the silence.

That is how it seems—but it is only how it seems. Once, while noticing that nobody was noticing, I felt ashamed at the lesson in Job's life. I still have a congregation of one in my wife, while poor Job was despised by his wife. Yet God was glorified by Job's faithfulness and is said to have pointed it out to Satan. Apparent losses were more than matched by the impact of that suffering life on the spirit realm. Also God met him before the finish line.

GETTING NEAR GOD

Scripture declares, "It is good to be near God" (Psalm 73:28). Down deep our hearts know it. But are we always aware when he is there? And exactly who are the ones with close-up privileges?

Is not the life of crucifixion, of which we have been speaking, often the way to this honored position? Being honored and humbled go well together. One afternoon, God taught me this lesson again.

With an especially heavy heart, I went out to the secluded back corner of our property that I have considered my prayer garden. I was desperate for God's renewing touch and so began praying earnestly.

As was so often the case, however, I heard the sound of the back door opening and of Jane's approaching footsteps. My solitude was over. But this time, rather than react with discouragement or irritation, a thought came to me: Why not seize this interruption as an opportunity?

I arose, welcomed my wife, and invited her to sit on the garden bench beside me. As she settled her head on my shoulder, the whole setting seemed one of prayer. God granted what I was praying for. He drew me near to him when I drew the weak, dependent, suffering one close to me.

As anyone who prays much knows, a major first issue in attempting to "get through" in prayer is that of establishing a proper alignment with the Father through the Lord Jesus Christ. All this seemed clear and right as we sat there together. Next, I read aloud Romans 8:28-39 and explained to Jane my need of prayer. She understood, at least, that her husband was hard-pressed in spirit. Because she was unable to pray, I launched into prayer, and God gave me at once the breakthrough I needed.

> For this is what the high and lofty One says—
> he who lives forever, whose name is holy:

> "I live in a high and holy place,
> but also with him who is contrite and lowly in spirit,
> to revive the spirit of the lowly
> and to revive the heart of the contrite."
> (Isaiah 57:15)

Those humbled to the dust lie near God's door. Experiences that are humiliating need not be degrading to one's spirit. Within the tough husk lies special sweetness. In Psalm 81:16 God speaks of providing "honey from the rock." It is wrong to expect much honey with no rock, and it is also wrong to settle for much rock with no honey.

Beating Up the Beautician

Probably few of the uninitiated could appreciate the thought, effort, patience, and persistence required to get a feisty dementia patient dressed and prepared for the day. My beloved sufferer over and again rejects and resists each piece of clothing. In fact, every day she refuses to allow the removal of her nightie in order to begin dressing. Then after some progress, when I turn to reach for the next article, she seizes upon the opportunity to put her nightwear back on.

The sight of the clothing on the foot of the bed is a call to arms for her. I have to be quick, creative, and resourceful in order to rescue the clothes from her and then get them on her. However, a seventy-seven-year-old husband down on his knees attempting to wash or dress his wife makes an inviting target for a quick shove or a solid punch to the head. Whenever this happened, alternative responses immediately rushed into my mind. Inner voices would call out to me, "Enough is enough! Can't she see you are on your knees in humble service to her? Shortcut through the misery; let her stay half-clad and smelly if that is what she wants." Then comes God's alternative—so different.

The quiet, inner voice of Jesus Christ, through the Spirit, comes to me: "My child, over years here and there you have resisted my efforts to wash your needy heart and life. How many times have I had to overcome your resistance to the fresh, clean spiritual apparel I have brought for you? Though done more slyly, you also have, on occasion, punched your Beautician! Who are you to wilt in self-pity and withdraw from the very schooling you so much need?"

RESTING IN PEACE ON THIS SIDE OF THE GRAVE

Friends insisted that I go through with my tentative plan to hire a lady to be with Jane a few hours in the middle of each day. Then a couple opened their home, providing an upstairs room overlooking an inlet of water where I could study, pray, and write this book.

I arrived extremely disoriented to begin my first hours away from Jane. She seemed in painful anxiety as I left and as the young stranger entered her life. I could not remember a time in the past year when we had been apart for so many hours.

Immersed in a strange mixture of joyful release, loneliness, and feelings of guilt, I climbed the stairs and shut myself in my new office. Next, I raised the blinds and savored the view. Just beyond the lawn was a footbridge over a stream, and beyond the bridge was a narrow neck of beach bordering an inlet of the Chesapeake Bay. Still looking out, I backed into my chair, opened my Bible at random, glanced down, and saw these words of Jesus to his wearied disciples: "Come with me by yourselves to a quiet place and get some rest" (Mark 6:31). (I have long opposed mishandling the Bible with what I call the "plop open and point" method of hearing from God. Given the powerful blessing of that moment, however, I quickly concluded that any good rule might have its exception!)

A similar experience occurred two months earlier when my quiet time of Bible reading at home was interrupted. Leaving the Scripture open on my desk, I hastened out to help Jane with bathroom proceedings. Then commenced the daily struggle to get her bathrobe on before breakfast. She threw off the robe in a burst of anger, so I retreated to the study to wait out the storm. I was startled when I resumed my reading in Psalm 119. Verse 165 was next: "Great peace have they who love your law, and nothing can make them stumble." Similar experiences with hymns on the radio have occurred over and again.

Two days ago, Jane made a flat, forceful, and final refusal to allow me to insert her dental plates. Speaking very plainly, and with an almost prophetic air, she said, "I won't be using those—*ever again*." The full realization hit me that this procedure is no longer to be my burden and that my remaining days of marriage will be spent with a toothless woman.

I will grant you that my pride was to the forefront, but I cared also for her dignity. At any rate, there I stood, leaning with both hands on the bathroom counter, in abject discouragement. At that moment, I became aware of music from our radio. The words being sung drew me back from the swamp of self-pity:

> Have we trials and temptations?
> Is there trouble anywhere?
> We should never be discouraged;
> Take it to the Lord in prayer.
> Can we find a friend so faithful,
> Who will all our sorrows share?
> Jesus knows our every weakness;
> Take it to the Lord in prayer.
> (from "What a Friend We Have in Jesus")

Our Lord Jesus Christ invites us in John 16:24 to turn our miseries into the joy of answered prayer. Prayer is the only way I know to conquer the impossibilities of caregiving.

Objectively, it moves mountains and changes things I can't budge, and it uncovers solutions I seem to miss. Subjectively, God lifts my drooping spirit, especially when I read and claim his own promises in Scripture. This divine gift of peace is instilled in the heart through the presence of the Holy Spirit.

MORE LESSONS FROM MY CROSS

Other lessons while on this cross have particularly probed my own heart, turning me from a downward to an upward look. Always a better view!

CHANGING SPIRITUAL ALIGNMENT BY MEANS OF ADVERSITY

Troubles check out our relationship with God, especially when our trials are intense and terminal. We are pressed to realign ourselves with the Power Source.

Racked by demands that seemed unthinkable yet destined to last for the rest of our life together, I begged God for release. No release came, but relief did. The familiar words of Proverbs 3:5-6 came alive to me. (How often does the gnarled hand of familiarity hide precious truth from us!) Directly, things changed. Now instead of being defeated by the grueling experiences, I witnessed—even participated in—my own private miracle.

I don't mean anything spectacular, but it is special nonetheless. Moment by moment, hour by hour, and day by day, as I am overburdened, I simply "plug into" the strength of the Almighty, which is always enough. That is what "trusting in the Lord" means to me. This transaction is accomplished in prayer, offered to the Father in Jesus' name, in accordance with John 14:13-14. Here is the workable alignment. On the one side, a man virtually overwhelmed and outclassed by his problems. On the other side, a God who can meet any need. Between stands Jesus Christ, the willing mediator. Problems practice us in prayer.

Two lethal mistakes stand close by: (1) thinking all is lost whenever the power drain is too heavy for my little battery and (2) thinking all is well because I have seen that God is able and willing to help. No, I must pray continually. God's supply meets my demand only as I pray.

KEEPING MY FACE TO THE WINDOW

After church services one Sunday, I thanked the considerate lady who had sat with Jane. Her reply taught me a lesson. "Your wife is always thinking of you and talking of you. She watches the door at the front through which you will enter to begin the service, saying, 'He's still in the study, but he will be out any moment.'"

Even at home, a closed door between us means agony for Jane. "May I open it just a little so I can see you?" is her plea. My prayer is, "Lord, help me to so love Jane—*and you*, longing for your presence and looking for your return."

On earlier occasions, while I was still engaged in daily pastoral duties, I would return home to see her anxious face at the window, looking for me to come. Then wrapping her arms around me, with tears brimming over, she would say with great joy, "Oh, God heard my prayer! I was praying and praying you would come. This is what I was talking and telling myself, what kind of a man you are and how I love you. I knew you would finally come!"

Oh, my Savior, help me to keep my face to the window "while we wait for the blessed hope—the glorious appearing of our great God and Savior, Jesus Christ" (Titus 2:13).

ESCAPING FROM TYRANNY TO A GRAND LIBERTY

My sad confession is that it took years of frustrations before I realized how tyrannical selfish desires are. Alzheimer's exposes, then mauls, the caregiver's personal interests. But wonderfully enough, what at first seems like a severe stripping, often turns out to be an avenue to freedom.

The daily discipline of having to distinguish between *what is right* and *what I only desire* squeezes me into this liberty. You must make a choice, however, to put to death sinful desire for the good of the suffering loved one. You virtually change wants.

Selfishness, though, rears its head again and again. It must be put to death daily. This is our personal crucifixion, according to Galatians 2:20, and must be accomplished in the Spirit's strength, through Christ.

Living Near the Well

Shall I get up and try again, or shall I give up? This question is unavoidable. Getting up again, and yet again, is the only way the caregiver can get through. (Besides, I never could figure out what "giving up" means and exactly how to do it.)

Conversely, the good hours tend to bring an unguarded euphoria at the pleasant relief. During such moments, I try to recall the sober warning of my good friend Robertson McQuilkin, who has many years of experience ministering to his wife who suffers from Alzheimer's. Cherish and try to remember the good times, he said, because they won't last—and when the really bad times come, don't overworry, because things will surely get worse! I have always been grateful for this admonition. It is indeed true.

But what does one do when those very real adversities clobber with such force that all meaningful married life seems at an end? Up come more deep groans, and out come more tears. That is how it is with me. I hurt for Jane and for me. But then I finally awaken and remember God's well. It's never dry.

In John 7:37 Jesus invites thirsty ones to drink freely from his supply. Verse 39 tells us that this drink is nothing less than the Holy Spirit. I read verse 38 with a peculiar delight. Here our Lord Jesus says to me, a bedraggled caregiver, that the supply is so adequate that I can overflow to my beloved wife and meet her need. I grant you that I don't feel like it can happen, but I pray with an open Bible, asking that this gracious filling be granted me yet again.

Living near the well and drawing from it in prayer throughout each day is a caregiving essential. Next, as mentioned in chapter 4, I must get up and practice God's two-step plan given to believers who are suffering: (1) commit oneself to God and (2) take the next step and continue to do the next right thing (1 Peter 4:19).

One other related lesson I'm learning is that prayer does not work mechanically, like an old gumball machine where you punch in your coin, hear the mechanism responding, and out comes your "answer." Prayer requires patience and endurance as you hold on in faith. Isn't that what Hebrews 10:36 is saying to us? "You need to persevere so that when you have done the will of God, you will receive what he has promised."

Running My Own Race

While writing down these thoughts, urgent interruptions deluged me. For example, there were cries for help to escape the clutches of "this evil person out here." I knew Jane was again confronting the one in the mirror. Shouting matches always follow.

I found myself again longing to discuss a thought or merely have an ordinary, rational conversation, instead of hearing the endless jabbering in nonsensical sounds and disjointed talking. Right then and there it came to me: here is my race; this is the way my course is laid out for me.

The moment I stopped looking at other smoother, more attractive tracks, it became much easier to run my own. The struggle ceased. I concluded that it is much harder to run looking sideways.

Nor is this a fatalistic cooperation with the unavoidable. Instead, it is a submission to a personal Lord—a willingness to run "the race marked out for us" (Hebrews 12:1; see also verses 2–12).

Avoiding the Looming Plague

Throughout the months prior to Jane's entry into the final phase of the disease, I was much engrossed in coping with the ordinary challenges while trying to keep my spiritual balance. Fortunately, a friend spoke a blunt word to me during this period. She said, "Beware of self-pity; it will destroy you!" Though inwardly I cried to hear a kinder word, what I heard was what I needed to hear, and deep down I knew it. The pity plague is ever near my door.

Afterward, God, in his own way, brought tender messages of solace. For example, I coaxed Jane across a busy parking lot, hobbling on my painful sprained ankle, only to be told in the store that the item I so much needed was sold out. Arriving back at our car, Jane jerked from my grasp and commenced yelling at her reflection in the door window. My spontaneous, no-help contribution was to order, "Don't! People will think we are fighting each other!"

When the combat ceased and Jane was seated and strapped in, I dragged myself around to the driver's side and sat for a time in physical pain and emotional stress. Then I turned on the car radio. Immediately, the words of the hymn "Be Still, My Soul" came out and met my need of the moment (just as these same words had come to me the morning after the especially upsetting event I described in chapter 5).

How much poorer I would be if God had opened my tight box and allowed me to escape! Whenever I look at all I might be missing, I am then looking outside the bounds of my box, which is devastating. In contrast, looking at all my supporting blessings draws me upward to see God in the box with me. That is how to hang on until relief comes. Self-pity makes me let go and miss the good.

Understanding a Wife's Wants

Startling indeed to me is the realization that things I now desire and understand are the very things I once was numb to and did not understand. I am referring to the things that my wife—and, I suppose, most other wives—would long for and, perhaps in vain, look for in her husband.

Frequently, at mealtime when I am chasing and persuading my wife to come to, or return to, the table, I seem to hear a familiar voice from my distant past begging me in the same way. Now I understand how it feels to see all one's kitchen efforts turn cold or melt.

If I could start married life again with Jane, how I would relish table conversation! What a delight to talk endlessly of precious memories! Would I not now appreciate all her care of the house? Indeed, if time could be rolled back and I had known then what I now know and feel, what a different husband I would be! Surely, I would assist her more, speak kind words of encouragement, and guard her from personal discouragement.

I still attempt to pray with Jane and share Bible phrases, but her mind cannot focus. Such activity was always a part of our life together. The devotion and love with which I now greet any opportunity go far beyond what I once was prepared for.

No tender words of appreciation or gratifying companionship can any longer be expected. Much has been exactly reversed. Things appear quite different when you look down from your cross. Many men will not see very deeply into their wives' hearts until the nails have fixed them to their cross.

LOOKING MORE DEEPLY AT ANGER

Experiences with dementia patients are undoubtedly similar to those other people endure, only more intense. This is a major thesis of this book. Things underscored, magnified, and intensified are more easily examined and explained. Alzheimer's disease makes each hangnail hurt a lot. Extremes are the routine. Take for example the matter of anger—I mean, getting red-hot mad. When one "goes after" a dementia patient, it makes no sense. Does it *ever* make sense to argue with one who does not have good sense?

Except for those welcome and tantalizing moments of exception, Alzheimer's patients live in a perpetual descent. Going after them in a rage not only invites calamity into that particular episode, but also lowers caregivers to the level of the patient. Higher ground is always abandoned in stooping to fight in the dingy cellars where our beloved "opponents" dwell. Well persons must not level with ill persons.

Under the magnifying glass of this ailment, two important truths about anger have been made clearer to me than ever before. First, yielding to irritation and anger removes the controls of caregiving from my hands. In any situation of marital tension, if the partner in the right abandons the light and enters the arena of anger to "get at" the other spouse, no one is left in the light and in control.

A case in point is when Jane is striding about in a rage and becoming aggressive. My only sensible option is to reach out in love. This means (as Scripture teaches) putting to death my native instincts and quietly saying over and again, "No matter what, Jane, I love you, and we're going to be happy together." I can usually manage a smile, and I touch her lovingly—even playfully—until finally she responds. Looking back, I can say that not one argument marred those moments when that was my approach.

A second illumination about anger (and how sweet it is to squeeze good juice from a bitter providence!) is that Alzheimer's, or any powerful negative pressure, is merely dredging up wrong responses. It does not plant them.

To avoid being misunderstood, let me agree that pent-up feelings often put people in bondage. But when it comes to anger, free expression is *not* the only alternative, nor is it the right one. Restraint and a healthy control are not the same as unhealthy, forced repression. Alzheimer's daily drubbing and steady barrages drive one who tends the patient to live in mean combat or else discover this truth.

Do not those who are despairing and shackled to some dark destiny find that life's lot tends to bring out long-hidden bitterness and anger that was assumed forever gone? Jesus taught that words (and other means of expressions) arise from the heart.

All of us must distinguish between the *occasion* and the *origin* of life's sinful expressions. Galling experience might occasion sinful anger, but it does not originate the sin. The trigger that fired the bullet did not load the gun. "All these evils come from inside and make a man 'unclean'" (Mark 7:23).

LEARNING TO LOVE

Will I never learn to love like God requires? Months have dragged into years, but the heavenly Instructor is tenacious. Besides, high fences encircle the school where love is being taught. I can't escape. In this school of experience, God is using Jane as his instrument to teach her slow-learning spouse what love is all about. She does so in three ways. Her *example* frequently shows love to me. Her *need* draws love from me. And even her *angry attacks* become a teaching tool, forcing me to love or give up.

Often, Jane sets before me a good example to follow of sincere, deep love. Like a beckoning hand poking through my black bewilderment, time and again I hear such words as, "Thank you. Thank you for taking care of me. You help me. You are the best I've ever seen. I love you so much." She melted my heart with all those words last night, even after being awakened from a sound sleep so I could slip on her protective briefs, which I had forgotten to attend to before bedtime.

"What's wrong with all these things?" she asked me a year or two ago. I knew she was referring to her fallen mental world, so I sought to give reassurance. "I know, honey, but it's my place now to help you. I'm your helper. That is what all men are supposed to be for their wives."

Not to be outdone, a few minutes later, she caught me staring off into space. "What is hurting you?" she inquired.

I answered her frankly. "I'm going to miss being a pastor."

"Don't give up, honey." Then a few minutes later she solemnly promised, "I'll help you any way I can."

Caught up one day in a flood of household duties, I paid little attention to the lonely lady who followed me from room to room. Our bed had to be changed. Two loads of laundry awaited. Breakfast, then the dishes, the dog, the trash; fix Jane's bathtub seat and clean the tub; prepare a not-so-good lunch and dinner; do the dishes and cleanup; take care of toilet duties and all the nightly tasks—Jane's dental care, undressing, bathing, tucking in bed. And many of these chores had to be performed against opposition.

Finally, a quiet, simple question penetrated my shrunken world. "You know what I want?"

"What is it that you want?

"You!"

"Oh, I'm so sorry. I've been too busy all day, I know." Instinctively, I probed a stock of possible reasons to offer but remained silent, reflecting on my behavior. One good thing about Alzheimer's is that you soon learn to scrap all excuses. No matter how they shine, all drop like lead. There I live in the squeeze between essential responsibilities and Jane's needs and longings.

Once I pleaded, in the face of her repeated interruptions, "Jane, I have to study."

"I know. That's why I'm going out." A moment later she was back with, "I don't want to hurt you. Don't be mad at me." A conscience, frequently pierced in such a manner, prepares one to learn more readily lessons in love.

Some months later, Jane expressed to me her anxieties with

unusual clarity. "I'm afraid I'm going to lose you. What would I do?"

"You know I love you. As God helps me, I will always be true to you. I really love you."

Later in bed that night, I was reading from Philippians 2:14, "Do everything without complaining or arguing." I recall at that moment looking down at her, lying beside me with her eyes wide open. She was looking up intently at my face.

"What are you doing? I thought you were asleep."

"I've got you!" is all she said.

Now I See!

*"Please, Daddy, where are you? Don't leave
me. I want to be with you. Oh, thank you!"*

—JANE, CLINGING TO ME IN A MOMENT OF
FEARFUL ANXIETY

"YOU ARE HEAVEN-SENT," I OFTEN SAID TO JANE WHEN WE WERE NEWLY-
weds. I meant that comment seriously. She brought an end to
a loneliness that had trailed me since I left my Tennessee home
for World War II duty aboard ship in the South Pacific.
Marriage was a matter of serious prayer before we met—she in
college and I in seminary. I knew at once that God had
answered my prayer.

In a far deeper way today, I know that Jane is heaven-sent.
As I have said, she is God's instrument for teaching me what
love is about. She shows me by her example, and she draws
me into love by her need. But also her frequent stubborn
resistance to all help, even her violent anger, has opened my
eyes to what seems to me to be love of a new order. Let me
explain.

I have begun to pity those who stride through life free and
unfettered. Love feelings came easily when my young wife was

so attractive to me. However, love limps badly when tethered only to attractions. Now that dementia has creased and bent her physically, broken her mentally, and distressed her emotionally, love is of a quality previously unknown to me. It was to help develop this love, I believe, that I was given the various lessons already shared. Capping all of them have been the insights shared here.

PRACTICAL, IMPOSSIBLE LOVE

It is the one who loves who must pay, and perhaps pay over and again. Or, putting it another way, the one who most needs you might most repel you. Then what? Where shall this deeper affection of which I speak be found? How do we get at it, practically?

Thankfully, it is not a matter of feelings. Nor of pity, which soon wilts. Nor of determination, as if the strong could somehow pull it off. The every-single-day battering is too much for those responses. Every day is a long time. We need help.

The apostle Paul uncovers in Romans 5:5 the secret for which we search: "God has poured out his love into our hearts by the Holy Spirit, whom he has given us." God is love (1 John 4:8, also verse 16). He is the Grand Source of every good gift, most especially of love. A believer's love for others arises in the will in concurrence and interaction with God's Spirit. We choose to love, and as we pray for our Lord's help to love, it comes to pass. God's well won't run dry. This love is an outflow from God through us and into the wasteland of need. As John said, "No one has ever seen God; but if we love one another, God lives in us and his love is made complete in us" (1 John 4:12).

God's means of sustaining me has been to grant me the capacity to love Jane, no matter what. It is rather like a private miracle, day by day and hour by hour. And it is happening within me. As I see and participate in this outflow of love toward Jane, I know surely that I did not generate it. (Though

I do beg for it in continual prayer.) My Lord has come very close—close enough to lift me back to my feet time after time.

Without doubt, I am no paragon of patience and humility, but when the stuffing has been knocked out of me, even I can sample the sweetness of 1 Peter 5:6: "Humble yourselves, therefore, under God's mighty hand, that he may lift you up in due time." This is how I see it, then. Because God's plan for my life is far more than I can handle, I am shut up to one, and only one, option. I must believe, pray, and cry out to him for understanding and strength to do that good will of God. Amen!

HIGH HEAVENS ABOVE DEEP WELLS

When I descended one night into another deep well of misery, I little expected to see something of heaven. (Around me every day, I see "free" people dancing in their dungeons of sin. I don't wish to live in such pleasant pollution, but I admit that suffering in God's will does hurt.) At my lowest, however, I saw further up. And it was good!

A cry in the night both awakened and informed me. The worst had happened. I rushed around to Jane's side of the bed and urged her toward the bathroom, trying to minimize the trail of urine across the carpet. The balance of the discharge pooled at our feet on the bathroom floor and mat. Quite naturally at that moment, I pleaded and coerced with all my energies to get her to be seated on the stool. She stayed standing.

My energies were next directed to holding her in place while I removed the soaked nightie and protected uninvolved areas. The moment of truth for me came while I was on my knees attempting to cleanse and remove Jane from the havoc. Her blows were landing on my unprotected head. My silent outcry was, "For *this* I get *that?*!"

Right then heaven suddenly opened over my deep well. I could see and hear—not with eyes and ears but with heart—

the Lord Jesus saying, "Now you know some of what I suffered for, and from, you. And what you did, you did with healthy brains!" It is clearer now that "God demonstrates his own love for us in this: While we were still sinners, Christ died for us" (Romans 5:8). Jesus' death was indeed for "God's enemies" (verse 10).

This same insight was underscored for me one morning while I was still serving as senior pastor. My secretary interrupted my studies to tell me that the volunteer caregiver at home was calling because of an emergency. Jane was refusing to finish dressing, so they could not go out to lunch as planned. "Get her topcoat on, and bring her to me," I suggested.

The plan fell apart at the church door. Slipping off the covering cloak, Jane strode into the hallway of the office wing dressed as she was at home: little nightie with two skirts and a pair of slacks underneath. I stepped from my office at the opposite end of the passage. What a pitiful sight she was, standing there at the far end of the hall, alone, unprotected, exposed! All the church's administrative and pastoral offices open on that busy hallway. It seemed a mile long as I rushed to meet her.

Being so intent on gathering Jane into my arms and shielding her from view, I was not conscious of those around. I drew her directly into my office. There in safety and seclusion, I held her until she understood that all was well.

My understanding also opened. I saw it clearly. The Lord Jesus had rushed to my aid and, bearing my shame and sin, he now shields me from all accusation. He shows more love to his Bride than I could ever show to mine.

SWEETEST FROM THE BITTEREST

How is it that those engulfed in God's hard and bitter providence often stand so near to his gentle and sweet presence? Some months back, the answer to this riddle came to me like fresh sunrays through my dreary clouds. I was reading in the Bible at Proverbs 1:23: "If you had responded to my rebuke, I would have poured out my heart to you and made my thoughts known to you."

Consider how singular are the lessons to be learned when one is under the discipline of divine wisdom. It is important, therefore, that the tested one not be paralyzed or become rebellious in such dealings. The heart of the Almighty wants to open to the heart of the aching.

Now I see, more than ever, that suffering believers are held near the heart of the loving Father who wields the rod. The wounded Shepherd cares for his wounded sheep. I must simply step out of the grief and senseless confusion of Alzheimer's and cast my sorrows on the One who bore my sins.

Jane's Prayers and Prophecies

"I think we will know . . . at the right time."
—JANE, SEEING MY CONCERN OVER THE
FUTURE AFTER RESIGNING MY PASTORATE

As far as I can tell, Jane has prayed her last out-loud prayer on earth and has spoken her final spiritual message. Though the candle in her soul's window outlasted other special lights from within her, it flickered and went out even as I beheld it. Feelings of both pain and privilege laid hold of me.

Before I share what Jane prayed and prophesied in those final utterances, I want to relate what I heard her pray and preach, as it were, over the last two years when I carefully recorded each word on the ever-present notepads. Then I will share what I learned standing in her last light.

I picture my beloved wife in the grip of this disease as a city overpowered by a devastating storm. The town buckles under the onslaught. Viewed from a distance, one might see entire sections lose power and yield to the darkness, first this subdivision and then that one. So it has been with Jane's inner life.

123

My record represents the ultimate flooding of the city, the onset of Alzheimer's final phase.

WORDS

Most of these little messages from Jane came unexpectedly, often arising during periods of confusion and meaningless talk. Some came like a flash of prophetic fire thrust directly at me or spoken Godward, while others were perhaps only talk with herself. In all, there were touches of tenderness and, not infrequently, an arresting authority about them. Here are a few assorted admonitions directed to me.

PROPHETIC WORDS AIMED AT ME

"Just Ask God . . . "

An insight into how a once-lively spiritual life fights for its breath in this final phase came to me recently. Jane was wandering back and forth through the house when she entered the room where I was. With emphasis and clarity, she said, "Just ask God himself to give us the help we need."

"That's a good idea; why don't we do it now?"

"Do what?"

"Let's pray and ask God himself to give us the help we need," I said, being careful to use her exact words. That failed to trigger her memory, but a flash of insight eased my frustration. I saw it clearly: Jane's spiritual life was preserved in wholeness, but her damaged brain blocked all but occasional, and treasured, manifestations.

A Benediction

A day of crisis for us came in late November of 1998. Having resigned weeks earlier, I preached my final sermon. That afternoon, I asked Jane to sit beside me. I tried to convey to her that I was no longer pastoring and that I felt a great need for us to pray together. Over and again I urged her to pray, to no avail.

With a heavy sigh, I did the praying.

In the middle of my telling God of our helpless uncertainty as to the future, she interrupted my labored prayer and spoke a significant sentence as plainly as anyone might say it: "I think we will really know . . . at the right time."

Our Worst Sunday

Among Jane's heartening words to me, none shone brighter than those she spoke at the end of our worst Sunday. We had been invited to dinner in a nearby restaurant, where Jane used the occasion to launch some of her most fiery missiles. "Shut up and leave this place!" she loudly confronted her reflection in the salad bar mirror. I tried to explain things to a shocked lady standing there. Back at our table, there was no peace. A nonstop stream of insults and inappropriate talk poured from her lips. At our evening service, nothing could curb her interruptions, so Jane was escorted out, while I continued to speak to those not distracted.

My hope of arriving home that night to a bit of peace was quickly dashed. In our absence our dog had vomited on the carpet and walked through the mess. To my utter dismay, at midnight, when I had barely finished the cleanup, my wife had a toilet accident.

After she was cleaned up and I was again on my knees working on the floors, Jane spoke beautifully, "Honey, we have had such a good life—all these years. God has been good to us."

Later in bed a quiet, reassuring voice called to me, "Remember, I'm right here if you need any help."

A Full Night and Next Morning

A lengthy episode that began in the middle of the night allowed me to view the pure stream of Jane's love, now so cluttered and covered by the disease. The preceding bedtime had been anything but easy, with Jane resisting undressing and preparing for bed. At 1:30 A.M. she was up and complaining of stomach pains. Next, "Is it okay if I take a bath?" (This was a couple years back in history when she could partly bathe herself.) Grudgingly, I prepared the bath water.

After her bath, I noticed she had her daytime clothes in hand, so I reminded her that it was still night and that she must return to bed. With obvious frustration she acquiesced, only to awaken soon with more cramps. After another hour or two of my "doctoring," we—or at least, I—fell asleep.

Then, "Honey, come see the . . . you know . . . bright in the heavens!" In great excitement, my wife stood at the window enjoying the first rays of the sunrise. I did not greet that dawn with singing. Rather, "Jane, you don't have many responsibilities today, but I do, and I need rest."

Before sleep could again bring its quiet, I heard a very faint whisper. Jane reached over to better cover me with the blanket, saying under her breath, "I did not mean harm; I was trying to help."

That ended my sleepiness. With a pierced conscience, I arose to greet the new day. Another such chastening awaited me later that morning. After another series of vexing sessions, I lapsed into feelings of self-pity. In this gray mood, I stood in the kitchen trying to decide what to do about breakfast.

Then came Jane. Positioning herself near me, she stood quite still examining a card she had received. In silence she stood there, looking at the card. Instantly, I knew what she was doing. That was the birthday card I had given her recently. Therein I had written of my undying, no-matter-what love. Then she spoke.

"I was just reading this again. I like it." She need not say more; I rededicated myself at once. Our breakfast was a happy one. Napkins, water, and most amenities were missing, and we had no milk on hand for cereal or coffee. But we were happy being together. Looking at her childlike and innocent expression, a thought overcame all else: "God helping me, I will endure anything to care for and protect you."

Other Prophetic Words to Me

- "I'm still here; I need you, too!" (spoken after catching me looking off into space with a worried expression). Later that evening she came to my study and pressed me wisely, "Are you coming? I think you should leave all that and come to bed."

- "I like to have you. I only have you for a few more days." (This one sure gave me cause for pause!)

- "I am a person, too, you know" (in response to my impatience).

- "Everyone has to do some thing—even if it is wrong." (Jane meant "wrong" here in the sense of "mistaken" or "incorrect." I had just stopped her from doing something that I feared might be harmful to her. Her words were spoken in quiet earnestness and obviously meant, "Don't stifle me by overcontrol.")

- "Just remember who you *aren't*."

- "Tell me what really comes into your heart" (Jane's effort to know what I was thinking and truly feeling).

- "Well, the world is still here" (spoken with a casual, in-case-you-hadn't-noticed-it attitude). Jane simmered me down with those half-dozen words at a time when I was thoroughly exasperated with her, when she was insisting on bringing to me the towel used to wipe the dog's muddy feet. Her quiet few words reminded me how useless it is to react to any such thing as if it is earth shaking, for lo! the earth still stands. (The apostle said the same thing in Philippians 4:5-7.)

- "Thanks for God giving me such a good man who tells me things I never knew." (In reality, I am the one in school.)

- "You know, I think God has you just where . . . in just the right place."

GENERAL SAYINGS

On several other occasions during the past months, Jane—in spite of everything that Alzheimer's has thrown up against her—has revealed her heart toward God, me, and even life in general. Overall, I consider all these expressions remarkable, given they were spoken by a mother who could no longer recognize the names of her own children. Here are some more general ones.

- "I am so happy to be happy!"
- "You know what? I sure do love God! I'm so glad he is there."
- "All this that God has given us shows us the way we should go and be" (spoken while seated in our den and surveying gifts from friends on the table, mantle, and walls). Another time Jane said, "Harold, God has been good to us with so many blessings!" (As we followed this exclamation with prayer, she was able to recount God's blessings to us over many years, even naming material things throughout our home.)
- "Look! Look at what God is doing!" (standing at the window during a storm).
- "I wish I could see our home—our real home." (I asked if Jane meant Rhode Island, where we used to live, among our children. Receiving no reply, I inquired further, "Do you mean heaven?" "Uh-huh," she answered.)
- "God has so much on his heart!"
- "Look at all God has made!" (said outdoors). At another time she regarded something in nature and said, "That really presses me in my heart."
- "We are the best [blessed] ones. God did it. Wonderful!"
- "I can see where I am going" (looking up in the sky).
- "I only have a little while to live. I want to be with my father and mother."
- "God is there in the heavens. Thank you! Thank you!" (looking out the kitchen window).

PRAYERS

The reaching up of any soul to God is a sensitive, special matter. How much more the struggles of one with Alzheimer's to maintain contact with her Father in heaven!

MORE IN THE HEART THAN MEETS THE EAR

A Prayerful "I Love You"

I would frequently assist her, quietly and gently, to begin to pray. On a Sunday afternoon several months ago, we were seated in our living room making an effort to worship together. I read several verses of Scripture, with a number of her interruptions, and led up to our time of prayer. I very much wished to hear her pray again.

"Now, you pray first, and I will pray next," I proposed. Instead, she said, "Do you see what I see?" She admiringly held up her wedding band, and I assured her of my love. After more of my urging, she began a prayer, but abruptly broke it off after only several words. Next came a stream of unintelligible words and syllables. I promptly prayed our closing prayer.

Again she held up the ring to the light and said with enthusiasm, "You know what? I really, really love you." Finally, it dawned on me that for God's broken child, it is my privilege to stand in for the Lord Jesus. So we ended our worship session rehearsing God's love in giving Christ and also in giving us to each other, for the past half-century.

Incidentally, the text I had read for us included Jeremiah 31:3: "The LORD appeared to us in the past, saying: 'I have loved you with an everlasting love; I have drawn you with loving-kindness.'"

A Painting of Jesus

Jane stood looking in the door of a small room in our home that had a favorite picture on the wall. "You know what I like best in this room?"

"Yes. You like the painting of Jesus knocking at the door."

Tears welled in her eyes as she exclaimed, "He has such good things in his heart!" The presence of Christ seemed very real to us both, so I offered prayer as we stood there in the doorway. For a time it was a regular stop in her wanderings about the house, and she was happiest if I came and commented on the scene.

Hoping to deepen her worship, I observed that she did not often speak of Jesus Christ anymore but referred only to God. Her response was immediate and strong: *"I do! I do all the time — in my heart!"*

PRAYERS EXPRESSED

On one occasion Jane reported spontaneously to me, "I was just thanking God for making me so happy today." As time went on, however, all her praying shut down except at meal-time. The familiar routine of table grace made it easier for her mind to engage and prayer to begin. In all, the prayers she did utter were offered with an earnest reverence and couched in such words that I could scarcely believe my ears. Here are some that I managed to get in writing. The list begins after the disease had progressed for several years and is presented in chronological order. The earlier prayers were of course better expressed, but the heart is the same throughout.

- "Help him not to be so aware of himself. You are the One who accomplishes all things. We praise you, O Lord" (Jane's prayer for her needy husband).
- "Father, I thank you for giving me yet a place. I know I can no longer take on things, but I pray that you will be gracious to me and that I can honor you and be faithful. I trust you, Lord, and I love you. Thank you for your Son sent to be our Savior."
- "Thank you for your kindness to me in helping me to settle down and not be worried over whether I do each thing just

right. And I especially thank you for the gracious way the women of the church receive me—and the gentle men of the church. You are good to give us a day such as this and a place to meet and worship you." (Prayed at church in my study, after Jane had "survived" the early worship service.)

- "O Lord, please send one of your angels to watch over me, and stand with me, and help me find my way this morning in the service" (also prayed at church, as Jane looked with great anxiety toward having to enter the sanctuary door where the congregation was seated).

- "O Lord, thank you for Harold that he is willing to hold on. I thank you that he does not give up but keeps me, and I love him with all my heart" (prayed a year later, after much coaxing; she turned in my direction as she prayed these words).

- "Father, we look up to heaven. You are over all the world, and the world. We thank you for all the good you do. We are so grandful to you. Amen."

- "Our Father, thank you for all the wonderful things you have given us from your home. Thank you. And thank you for all you have done. And I do love you. Amen."

- "Our Father, thank you that you are so gracious and good, and especially that we can love each other. Amen."

- "Thank you for all the things in our lives we have seen from you. And, just think what it's like for those who don't know any of this!"

One particularly bad day, Jane looked out the window and referred to the dog as "our children outside." In spite of her mental state, I repeatedly asked her to pray at our noon meal. Finally, she did, with tears of joy. "Thank you for all you give to those who are in your heart and are your children. And I love you. Boy! I love you! I really do love you! Oh, I love you! I love you!"

In the fall of 1999 I did not know that I was about to hear Jane's next-to-last prayer. She had been silent during mealtime prayer for nearly a month. We were finishing another "worst week," and I urged her to pray. Her little prayer took me by surprise and sent me afterward scurrying from the table to write it down. It came about when I asked yet again, "Will you pray, please, and thank the Lord for this food?" She replied firmly, "Yes, I will." Then she said, "Father, I thank you as well for that time when I first looked up to you and into your heart. Thank you! Amen."

THE LAST LIGHT

Ever since first meeting Jane I have been impressed by the way she prays. Over the years, as we prayed together daily and battled our way through many a crisis, I personally experienced remarkable uplift from hearing her address God during her particularly solemn and powerful prayers. Yet I could never seem to grasp what it was about her prayers that made them seem so special.

Now I think I know; the afternoon of that last prayer it was understandable to me. Her prayers are so stirring because of their deep reverence for the Almighty and her strong confidence that prayer is nothing less than our way of relating to him and God's way of getting his work done. In recent days her prayers had become increasingly limited and childlike, yet even these carried something of the atmosphere of former years.

Hearing Jane pray one more time—at one o'clock in the afternoon of December 8, 1999—touched me beyond what any words of mine could ever convey. She had not prayed with me for weeks, and I had ceased trying to persuade her. Much of the time, she did not comprehend what was being requested. Usually, her only response was nonsensical talk. On other occasions she could understand only well enough to say, "No, *you.*" Sensing her confusion, as desire struggled against both the dimness of thought and the inability to get her faculties to perform, I would pray each time for both of us.

On this date I felt in my heart that I ought to try once

more. The usual babbling greeted my first efforts. I tried yet again. Jane became completely quiet, and a look familiar to me came over her face—an expression of serious intent. Then she began the one dozen words of her final prayer:

Father in heaven,
I thank you
For what you have made us.

That is all she said, before her mind skipped to other things. Suddenly, the light she yielded seemed to dawn on me. All this—these years of trial—are for our good, to make us what God wants us to be!

A month later—on Sunday, January 23, 2000—Jane gave me a final prophetic word. If any more of these coherent sayings come, fine, but I do not expect them. This little prophecy, which ties in with her final prayer, seems to be the concluding illumination on our years of confusion.

That special Sunday was anything but special in its beginning. Getting Jane dressed was a contest. She stood at the breakfast table with only one arm in her dangling blouse and her arms and hands loaded with stuffed animals, greeting cards, paper napkins, and the like. I could not coax her to eat or to finish dressing. She lashed out at me with fists and angry words, warning of unseen evil on the prowl around us.

A few minutes later she agreed to go to the bathroom. I noticed again that she did not know the way, although we live in a small one-level home. Suddenly she stood still in the middle of the room and, with a faint smile, spoke the following words as clearly as any of earlier years.

God is really giving us
A chance to be
Somebody nice.

From my heart, and without reservations, I say, Amen!

How could I, my faithful reader, pour out in words what these years with God's afflicted child Jane have meant to me? I have tried, and you have listened. May God in turn add his glow to each life.

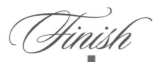

My Confessions and Tribute to Jane

"Do you think I will ever have such a glow?"

—JANE, SAID EARLY IN OUR MARRIAGE
ABOUT A GODLY WOMAN SHE ADMIRED

JANE, MY DEAR WIFE, I HAVE MANY TIMES OVER MANY YEARS SPOKEN words of love to you. I realize you no longer fully understand my efforts, though sometimes you say a polite "Thank you" or "Me, too." Now I put this tribute in words you will never read.

Here I am, more than ever before, pouring out my love for you at a time when you can no longer comprehend. I know that, if you could, you would forgive me for the things I have mentioned in this book. How I wish you could! You were so right when, as I recounted at the start, you predicted that God would one day humble me beyond anything I had ever known. I hope that I am passing the course.

Remember when we were newlyweds? You had returned from a meeting for women of the church and were deeply impressed with the mature lady who led the study. With admiration you described her as a "gracious and godly woman." Longingly, you asked me, "Do you think I will ever have such a glow?"

That radiance had already begun, I knew, and—in an almost-prophecy—I told you so. You hardly accepted what I said then, nor were you fully convinced when I reiterated it at other times. I wish I had tried harder. Indeed, the godly glow today is so strong and genuine that it frequently penetrates the clouds of your disease. I revere what God has done.

In lectures, writings, and personal exhortations I have been taught much by many. But you have changed my life. You worked some in my head but much in my heart. I am grateful to be free from the cocoons in which I struggled.

For many a year, you served our family, and me in particular. Beyond that, you labored actively with me in ministry for half a century. What I render to you now is small in comparison. I am thankful that God is giving me the strength to do it.

Several times in recent months, I could tell you were concerned for my welfare. You seemed to understand that I was in over my head endeavoring to be a homemaker and also to care for you. Yet when Peter walked on water toward Jesus, it did not matter how deep the water was so long as he was above it. Even when he was sinking, there was no danger because he had the good sense to call out to Jesus. I am well practiced in making Peter's desperate plea, "Lord, save me!" (Matthew 14:30). Alzheimer's waves are too much for any person. Good swimmers struggle more; I'm learning to call and rest. The Lord Jesus is bringing me into his new world where swimmers sink and sinkers float.

You and I have over and again committed ourselves to these truths. We were saved from our sin by Christ's blood-offering on the cross, and by that same Good News we are enabled to stand steady and live for God, exactly as Scripture says in 1 Corinthians 15:1-4: saved and sustained by the same Savior.

I am not sure you ever really understood what I meant when I described you to others as the world's most unusual woman. I always admired you because you were deep and different—different in the sense of special. "A wife of noble character is her husband's crown" (Proverbs 12:4). Thanks for the crown.

Amen.

About the Author

After half a century of pastoral experience, Harold Burchett has been forced to dig to a new level of personal life and ministry. No longer caring for a large congregation, he is daily striving to dress, give personal care, and offer spiritual nurture to one who is drifting ever deeper into the darkness of dementia. As homemaker and major caregiver for his wife, Jane, an Alzheimer's patient, he is more often cleaning up accidents in the bathroom than performing public duties. He testifies that new insights into Scripture and a more real fellowship with the Lord have resulted from the dark days and long nights. These encouragements have kept despair at bay. *Last Light* was produced during the pitch of this privately fought battle as Jane uttered her last prayers and final words of admonition to her husband. Burchett's other ministries still carry a dedication to discipling and leadership training and a concern for a spiritual awakening in the churches.

A Note From the Author: At this writing, Jane's decline continues at about the same rate, which means more of Alzheimer's and less of Jane, day by day. Though she now asks, "Who are you?" she never relates to me as a stranger. In all, the problems simply keep increasing—likewise God's grace.

MORE INSPIRATIONAL BOOKS FILLED WITH HOPE AND ENCOURAGEMENT.

The Message: New Testament Psalms and Proverbs

Experience the life-changing power of the New Testament, the vibrant passion of the Psalms, and the rich, practical wisdom of Proverbs.
(Eugene H. Peterson)

The Message Promise Book

This pocket-size book arranges passages from *The Message* by topic, making it easy to find out what God's Word says about a particular subject.
(Eugene H. Peterson)

Restore My Soul

This guide provides gentle help for those looking to put back together the pieces of a life shattered by loss.
(Lorraine Peterson)

To Walk and Not Grow Weary

Renew your strength by examining the lives of twelve biblical characters who triumphed in depressing circumstances.
(Fran Sciacca)

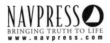